SpringerBriefs in Public Health

For further volumes:
http://www.springer.com/series/10138

Duncan Dartrey Adams
Christopher Dartrey Adams

Autoimmune Disease

Pathogenesis, Genetics, Immunotherapy, Prophylaxis and Principles for Organ Transplantation

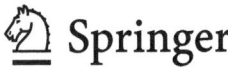 Springer

Duncan Dartrey Adams
Faculty of Medicine
University of Otago
Dunedin
New Zealand

Christopher Dartrey Adams
Analogue Digital Instruments
Dunedin
New Zealand

ISSN 2192-3698   ISSN 2192-3701   (electronic)
ISBN 978-94-007-6936-6   ISBN 978-94-007-6937-3   (eBook)
DOI 10.1007/978-94-007-6937-3
Springer Dordrecht Heidelberg New York London

Library of Congress Control Number: 2013940952

Printed on acid-free paper

Springer is part of Springer Science+Business Media (www.springer.com)

This book is dedicated to Sir Charles Hercus
Dean of the Otago Medical School
1937–1958. He fostered research

Charles Hercus was a brave, kind Viking whose
ancestors came from the Shetland Islands. After
serving with the New Zealand Army Medical Corps
on Gallipoli in World War 1, Colonel Hercus DSO
became concurrently Professor of Bacteriology,
Professor of Preventive Medicine and Dean of the
Otago University Medical School, eventually being
knighted. Full of zeal for abolishing disease, Hercus
recruited the brilliant scientist HD Purves, with whom
he got rid of New Zealand's endemic goitre, and
Duncan Adams with whom he set in motion research
that has solved the pathogenesis and genetics of the
autoimmune diseases.

Foreword

Pathogenesis. This book describes how, in the 1900s, in the field of Medicine, the Jerne-Burnet Forbidden Clone Theory and the Adams-Knight H Gene Theory, solved the pathogenesis and genetics of the autoimmune diseases and show how specific immunotherapy and prophylaxis can be developed.

Genetics. Building on the Forbidden Clone Theory, discovery of autoimmune anemia and lupus nephritis in Bielschowsky's NZB mice and Vladutiu and Rose's discovery that the MHC influences risk of autoimmune disease, Adams and Knight arrived at the H Gene Theory of the genetics of autoimmune disease. This states that histocompatibility antigens, major, minor, and H-Y (the male sex antigen), together with the V (variable region) genes for B and T lymphocytes, are the germ-line immune response genes, the genes that influence risk of autoimmune disease.

Microbial triggers. A major advance was Ebringer's discovery that a microbial trigger of rheumatoid arthritis is the bacterium *Proteus mirabilis*, with molecular demonstration of how a histocompatibility antigen can predispose to an autoimmune disease by preventing reaction with a similar antigen on the microbe, and so favour reaction with another antigen on the microbe that has similarity to an autoantigen at risk of being attacked by a forbidden clone arising by somatic mutations in multiplying lymphocytes.

Prophylaxis. The need for this exemplifies the importance of finding the microbial triggers for all the autoimmune diseases, so that they can be prevented by vaccination against their triggering microbes. Such prevention has happened with poliomyelitis vaccination, which has prevented post-poliomyelitis leg paralyses, which can now be seen to have been rare autoimmune complication of the virtually universal poliomyelitis virus infections.

Contents

1 Discovery. 1
  The Germ Theory of Disease 1
  Ehrlich's Side Chain Theory. 1
  Horror Autotoxicus 1
  Discovery of Autoimmune Disease 2
  Classification of Adverse Immune Reactions 2
  Synopsis of the Immunity System 3
  Therapy and Prophylaxis for the Infectious Diseases 3
  Autoimmune Disease. Steps in Discovery of its Existence,
  Pathogenesis, Genetics, Immunotherapy and Prophylaxis 4
  A Plague of Goitre in New Zealand. 4
  Kelly and Sneddon Discover Why Iodine Deficiency Occurs 5
  Hercus, Purves and Goitre in New Zealand 6
  Discovery of Antithyroid Drugs 7
  Solution of Pituitary Gland Cytology. 8
  Adams' Entry into the Research World 9
  Graves' Disease 10
  Radioactive Iodine. 11
  Thyroid Research with Radioactive Iodine 11
  Discovery of Long-Acting Thyroid Stimulator 12
  LATS Protector. 16
  A Letter from Deborah Doniach 16
  LATS Protector, the Specific Human Thyroid Stimulator. 16
  Exophthalmos. 18
  Neonatal Thyrotoxicosis. 18
  References 18

2 Pathogenesis 21
  Immune Tolerance. 21
    Nossal's Key Experiment. 21
    Discovery of the Structure of Antibody Molecules 22

Discovery of T and B Lymphocytes 23
   Types of T Lymphocytes (T Cells) 24
   Regulation of Immune Responses 25
   Suppressor T Cells as the Cause of the Autoimmune Diseases 26
   Loss of Suppressor T Cells does not Cause
   the Autoimmune Diseases 26
Solution of the Pathogenesis of Autoimmune Disease 26
   Jerne's Selection Theory of the Immune Response 26
   The Immunological Clone 27
   Burnet's Clonal Selection Theory of the Immune Response 27
   Burnet's Forbidden Clone Theory of Autoimmune Disease 27
   Cytotoxic T Cell Forbidden Clones 28
   Graves' Disease, a Paradigm for Autoimmune Disease 28
   Pathogenic Forbidden Clones; Discovered Ones
   and Ones Awaiting Discovery......................... 30
References 30

3   Genetics. 33
The Familial Aggregation............................... 33
Discovery of the Histocompatibility System 33
The Major Histocompatibility Complex 34
Involvement of the MHC in Autoimmune Disease 34
Functions of the Major Histocompatibility Complex 34
Benacerraf and McDevitt's Mistake........................ 36
Solution of the Genetics of Autoimmune Disease;
The H Gene Theory. 36
   The H Gene Theory of Inheritance of Autoimmune Disease. 37
   The Alternative Clonal Development Concept 37
   Confirmation at the Molecular Level..................... 37
   Immune Response Genes 38
A Fourth Gene Category for McKusick's Catalogue 38
   Schizophrenia..................................... 38
   The Knight Model of Schizophrenia 39
References 40

4   Microbial Triggers. 43
Information from Sequencing Antigens on Bacteria
that Trigger Autoimmune Diseases 44
   How Histocompatibility Antigens Predispose to
   Autoimmune Diseases 45
Four Laws of Autoimmunity.............................. 46
References 48

5   **Immunotherapy**   49
    Generalised Immune Suppression   49
    Immune Ablation and Autologous Bone Marrow Cell Restoration. . . .   49
    Selective Destruction of Forbidden Clones   50
    References   51

6   **Prophylaxis**   53
    Post-Measles Encephalomyelitis and Ender's Measles Vaccine   53
    The Poliomyelitis Epidemics.   53
    Was the Paralysis a Rare Autoimmune Complication
    of Universal Virus Infection?   54
    The Lead in Prophylaxis Given by the Polio Vaccines.   54
    Finding Microbial Triggers.   54
    Possible Therapy by Vaccination against Microbial Triggers   54
    References   55

7   **Transplantation**   57
    References   57

Prologue

"The history of scientific and technical discovery teaches us that the human race is poor in independent thinking and creative imagination. Even when the external and scientific requirements for the birth of an idea have long been present, it generally needs an external stimulus to make it actually happen; man has, so to speak, to stumble right up against the thing before the idea comes [1]."

Albert Einstein

Reference

1. Einstein A. Essays in science. New York: Philosophical Library Inc.: 1934. p. 92

Chapter 1
Discovery

The Germ Theory of Disease

Louis Pasteur revolutionised medicine with his epochal Germ Theory of Disease [1].

The great host of infectious diseases, with their aetiology at last discovered, were soon substantially conquered. Vaccinations provided prophylaxis and antibiotics, therapy. Additionally, freed of inevitable wound infection, modern surgery was made possible, led by Joseph Lister [2]. Additionally, Pasteur's great discovery revealed the existence of the immunity system, for defence against diseases caused by bacteria, viruses and worms.

Ehrlich's Side Chain Theory

After the discovery of antibodies, Paul Ehrlich [3] observed that goats injected with red blood corpuscles from other goats made specific antibodies against them and after a second injection the antibody response was increased. He correctly concluded that antibodies had "side chains" that reacted with specific antigens and that the cells possessing specific side chains increased in number after contact with a complementary antigen. Today, Ehrlich's side chains are confirmed as real, being the antigen receptor fraction of antibody molecules, as described below.

Horror Autotoxicus

Before World War 1, search for autoimmune disease was a common medical research activity, according to Dr Walter Griesbach, a Hamburg physician exiled to New Zealand by the Nazis. But after that terrible war had destroyed a whole generation of men, the scant survivors mistakenly taught that Paul Ehrlich had proved that autoimmunity never happens, so called "horror autotoxicus."

D. D. Adams and C. D. Adams, *Autoimmune Disease*,
SpringerBriefs in Public Health, DOI: 10.1007/978-94-007-6937-3_1,
© The Author(s) 2013

This mistake blocked the discovery of autoimmunity for decades. In reality, with Morgenroth, Ehrlich was able to cause goats to produce antibodies by injecting them with red blood cells of other goats, but attempts to immunize goats against their own red cells did not succeed (Ehrlich and Morenroth 1901) [3]. Ehrlich correctly concluded that animals will not normally make autoantibodies against their own tissues (immune tolerance), but that "possible failure of the internal regulation of immune processes might be the explanation of many disease phenomena."(Ehrlich and Morgenroth 1900) [3].

Discovery of Autoimmune Disease

The first to break the prevailing false dogma of "Horror autotoxicus" was the haematologist Dameshek [4], who recognised the existence in people of autoimmune haemolytic anaemia. This was followed by Witebsky and Rose [5], who induced autoimmune thyroiditis in rabbits, using Freund's adjuvants [6] which had enabled him to cause autoimmune destruction of testes in guinea pigs by prolonging antigenic stimuli to allow time for somatic mutations in responding lymphocytes. Doniach and Roitt [7] discovered autoantibodies to thyroglobulin in people. Then came discovery by Adams and Purves [8–10] of the thyroid-stimulating autoantibodies that cause thyrotoxicosis by accidentally reacting with the thyroid gland's receptor for thyrotrophic hormone from the pituitary gland.

Classification of Adverse Immune Reactions

During the decades' long reign of "horror autotoxicus", Coombs and Gell [11] published a classification of adverse immune reactions. Still believing that autoimmunity never happens, they used the term "**hyper-**sensitivity" for what is **mal-**sensitivity, and made a false classification of types of immune reactions that excluded autoimmunity. The independent demonstration of autoimmunity in four different laboratories [4–10] made Coombs and Gell's classification obviously wrong, yet it lingered on for decades [12] as an inhibition to clarity of thought.

Table 1.1 shows a valid classification of adverse immune reactions [13].

Type I is allergy and anaphylaxis, a worm-defence system, reacting to non-worm antigens.

Type II is serum sickness, due to excessive quantities of antigen, first seen following passive immunisation with horse antiserum to tetanus or rabies.

Type III is autoimmunity, divided into

Type III B caused by forbidden clones of B (bone marrow derived) lymphocytes and Type III T caused by forbidden clones of T (thymus derived) lymphocytes.

Table 1.1 Classification of immune reactions causing disease

Type I. Allergy and anaphylaxis

Gut worm-defence mechanism reacting to non-worm antigens [41, 42]

Fault: a B lymphocyte IgE clone reactive with an allergen

e.g. hay fever, anaphylaxis, gut allergy, skin allergy

Type II. Serum sickness and immune complex disease

Fault: excessive quantity of antigen

This swamps complement-neutralising mechanisms, leading to complement-mediated damage. Anti-microbial immune defense is designed to cope with picogram quantities of antigen, not milligrams of horse serum protein nor micrograms of released intra-cellular protein, such as nuclei [43, 44]

e.g. serum sickness following passive immunization against diphtheria toxin with horse serum, systemic lupus erythaematosus, lupus nephritis

Type III. Autoimmunity

Fault: forbidden clones, which are anti-microbial lymphocyte clones with accidental host-antigen specificity, arising from unlucky somatic mutations in their lymphocyte V genes [13, 38]

Type III B. Diseases caused by B lymphocyte forbidden clones:

e.g. Graves' disease [10], myasthenia gravis [45], rheumatoid arthritis [46]

Type III T. Diseases caused by T lymphocyte forbidden clones:

e.g. Diabetes Type 1 [47, 48], diabetic retinopathy [49, 50], experimental autoimmune encephalomyelitis [51] and presumptively Addison's disease, hypoparathyroidism, and other autoimmune diseases with specific parenchymal cell destruction [43]

Sir Ronald Bodley-Scott, President of the Royal College of Physicians, wisely stated that the last two decades of the 1800s are yet to be surpassed in medical research achievement.

Synopsis of the Immunity System

In the blood, there are "formed elements", cells, as well as dissolved molecules that include gamma-gobulins, which are the antibodies.

Little red blood cells, full of haemoglobin, carry oxygen from our lungs to our tissues, to give us the energy for all our activities.

Little white blood cells (white soldiers) defend us from infection by gobbling up germs. They are visible under the microscope, with germs inside them.

Renegade white soldiers cause autoimmune diseases by attacking a part of our bodies, in mistake for a germ.

Therapy and Prophylaxis for the Infectious Diseases

Antibiotics, e.g., sulphadiazine, kill germs without being toxic to human tissues.

After World War 1, Alexander Fleming, seeking germ-killing agents for curing infected wounds, discovered **Penicillin,** made by the soil-inhabiting fungus

Penicillium notatum. It is active against many bacteria, including the dangerous gram-positive pathogens, streptococci, staphylococci, pneumococci and also the spirochetes, *Treponima pallidum,* that cause syphilis. Unfortunately, before this was known, the British Medical Research Council declined Fleming's research application for a chemist to purify penicillin, so it lay latent for many years.

Fortunately, the Australian doctor, Howard Florey, rigorously searching the literature for antibiotics for treating the wounded in World War II, came across Fleming's papers on penicillin. He recognized the importance of penicillin and succeeded in harnessing US industry to produce it in useable quantities for use towards the end of the war. Fleming and Florey shared the Nobel Prize for Medicine in 1945.

Many more antibiotics exist, all made by microbes to defend themselves against competing microbes. Some were discovered at sewer outlets, where human pathogenic microbes are present and their microbial competitors make substances to kill them.

Vaccines, made from killed or attenuated pathogenic bacteria or viruses, are used for active immunization, providing prophylaxis against infectious diseases, but often with a small risk of accidental autoimmune attack on the nervous system, called **encephalomyelitis.**

Autoimmune Disease. Steps in Discovery of its Existence, Pathogenesis, Genetics, Immunotherapy and Prophylaxis

Major steps in the research that has led to today's understanding of the autoimmune diseases and how to develop immunotherapy and prophylaxis for them, are described and summarised in Table 1.2

A Plague of Goitre in New Zealand

A consequence of its geological history is that New Zealand, like Switzerland, had endemic goitre, widespread occurrence of enlargement of the thyroid gland. This was studied by Hercus, Benson and Carter [14], who measured frequency of goitre all over New Zealand, relating this to the local iodine content of the soil. Endemic goitre is caused by deficiency of **iodine**, a trace element, needed by man and other animals because it is a component of thyroid hormone, which regulates our metabolism. Endemic goitre was also prevalent in Chile, another mountainous country, dominated by the great Andes Mountains.

Table 1.2 Autoimmune disease. Steps in discovery of its existence, pathogenesis, genetics, immunotherapy and prophylaxis

Graves, Basedow. Clinical recognition of thyrotoxicosis

Dameshek, Witebsky and Rose, Doniach and Roitt. Discovery of autoimmunity

Adams and Purves and Roitt. LATS protector. Receptor autoimmunity causes thyrotoxicosis

Haldane. Comprehension of tissue allo-antigens, the histocompatibility antigens

Mitchison. Discovery that allo-grafts are rejected by lymphoctes (T cells), not by antibodies

Gorer, Snell, Klein. Details of the histocompatibility system in mice

Dausset, Benaceraf, McDevitt, Bodmer. Details of the major histococompatibility system in man, where the antigens were designated human leukocyte antigens (HLA)

Terasaki. Huge effect of HLA B27 on risk of ankylosing spondylitis, triggering extensive study of effects of HLA antigens on risks of autoimmune diseases

Zinkernagel and Doherty. Viral peptides are presented to T cells on histocompatibility antigens

Adams. The explosive speed of viral replication makes involvement of histocompatibility antigens essential for defence against virus infection

Jerne. The *selection theory* of immune response. Antibodies are not constructed on a template. They are preformed and selected by antigen

Burnet. It is not antibodies that are selected, but the cells that make them. These cells are the lymphocytes, that exist as clones of cells with identical receptors for antigen, hence the clonal selection theory of immune response

Forbidden clones, arising by somatic mutation in V genes, cause autoimmune disease. Proven for Graves' disease by Knight et al.

Bielschowsky. The NZB inbred mouse develops autoimmune anaemia

Howie and Helyer. The (NZB × NZW)F1 hybrid mouse develops lupus nephritis

Knight and Adams. Three genes for lupus nephritis, leading to

Adams and Knight. The *H gene theory* of inheritance of autoimmune disease. Histocompatibility antigens, major, minor and HY (the male sex antigen), by deleting complementary new lymphocyte clones, police the immune repertoire, *protecting* from autoimmune diseases, with variably imperfect success

Kaplan. Total lymphoid irradiation with bone marrow reconstitution enables allograft acceptance and cure of autoimmune disease, a consequence of the Forbidden clone theory, as unlucky somatic mutations are unlikely to recur

Smith. Use of bacteriophage peptide display libraries could reveal undiscovered forbidden clones

Vassart and Dumont. Cloning of the Graves' disease auto-antigen

Adams and Knight. Recognition that cloned autoantigens could be attached to a cytotoxic moiety to make a therapeutic molecular complex for selectively destroying the forbidden clone, leaving the rest of the immune system intact

Ebringer. Discovery that *Proteus mirabilis* triggers rheumatoid arthritis and *Klebsiella pneumoniae* triggers ankylosing spondylitis

Adams, Knight and Ebringer. All autoimmune diseases have *microbial triggers*, therefore prevention of autoimmune diseases will come from finding and vaccinating against their microbial triggers

Kelly and Sneddon Discover Why Iodine Deficiency Occurs

The Chilean Government had the wisdom to set up the Chilean Iodine Educational Bureau, in London, employing two outstanding English chemists, FC Kelley, BSc, PhD, FRIC, and WW Snedden, MA, PhD, FRIC. In their classical book on

"Prevalence and geographical distribution of endemic goitre", these able scientists explain how iodine deficiency arises [15]. Iodine does not come from the weathering of rock. It is dissolved in the sea, from which it vaporizes by oxidation, to be deposited in soils by rain. From the soil, iodine is taken up by plants, from whence it comes to man, directly in vegetables and fruit, or indirectly through meat animals. Iodine takes a long time to build up in soils to the levels we need for manufacture of sufficient thyroid hormone. Geologically old soils, like those of England and France and the eastern United States, contain adequate iodine for human need, but the new soils of Switzerland, the Himalayas, Chile and New Zealand, where there has been geologically recent up-thrust of mountains, have not had time to accumulate adequate amounts of iodine to meet the needs of humans and other animals. This causes goitre, an enlargement of the thyroid gland, caused by increased secretion of thyroid-stimulating hormone from the pituitary gland, aimed at enabling the thyroid to absorb more iodine from the blood.

Hercus, Purves and Goitre in New Zealand

Charles Hercus (Fig. 1.1) was a brave, kind, Viking, whose ancestors came from the Shetland Islands. After serving with the New Zealand Army Medical Corps in Palestine and Gallipoli in Word War 1, Colonel Hercus DSO, became concurrently Professor of Bacteriology, Professor of Preventive Medicine and Dean of the Otago University Medical School, eventually being knighted. New Zealand in the 1920s was riddled with goitre, necessitating countless subtotal thyroidectomies for obstruction of the trachea and for hyperthyroidism. An extreme case of goitre is shown in Fig. 1.2, depicting a Maori lady in the 1920s. By the time of World War II, surgeons in New Zealand hospitals were busy, several times a week, cutting out goitres from the countless people who suffered hoarseness from pressure on the recurrent laryngeal nerve or suffocation from obstruction of the trachea. In the course of his efforts to abolish the goitre endemic, Hercus recruited the brilliant HD Purves (Fig. 1.3), who had Honours degrees in the basic sciences, physics and chemistry, Hercus encouraged him to undertake the medical course, including a period in general practice. Thus Purves acquired the great breadth of biological knowledge encompassed by medicine. Throughout his career Purves' active mind enabled him to keep up with the principles of science as they slowly advanced, a mental activity that gave him the continuing authority of an impeccable scientific foundation.

Unexpectedly, despite, the addition of iodine to domestic salt in New Zealand, goitres continued to occur. Purves discovered why [16]. After comparing urinary iodine excretion of New Zealanders with that of Samoans, who had no goitre, Purves iodised the salt used by the Dunedin Hospital nurses with a fly spray, increasing the amount until the nurses' urinary iodine excretion matched that of the Samoans. He found that the amount needed was one part of potassium iodide per 20,000 parts of sodium chloride. This was 10 times more than the ineffectual

Fig. 1.1 Sir Charles Hercus, Dean of the Otago Medical School, Dunedin, New Zealand. He fostered research, which got rid of hydatids and goitre and led to discovery of the autoimmune diseases

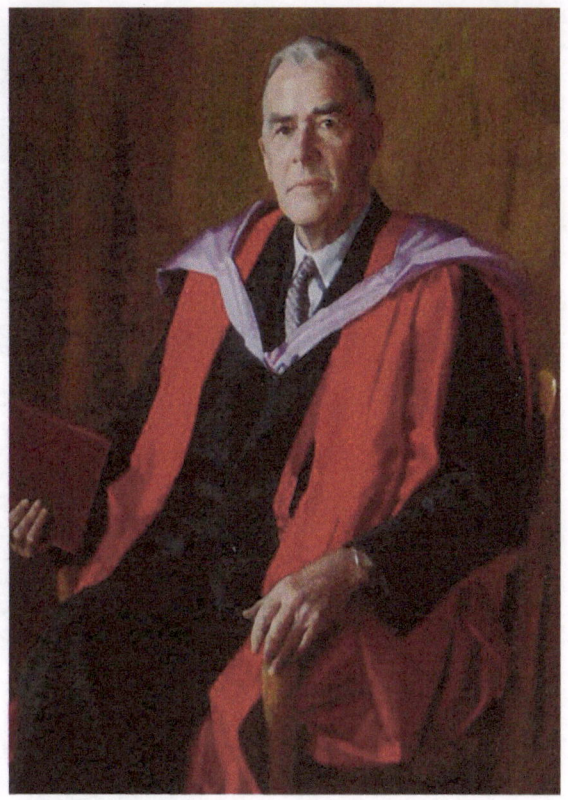

level previously used in New Zealand. Introduction of the new level in the early 1940s abolished New Zealand's goitre endemic. This successful prophylaxis has saved New Zealanders from thousands of subtotal thyroidectomies and from the birth of cretinous children.

Discovery of Antithyroid Drugs

Apart from iodine deficiency, Chesney, Clawson and Webster [17] discovered that thyroid hyperplasia could be caused by feeding rabbits cabbage diets. Exploring this, Kennedy and Purves found that brassica seed diets would cause goitre in rats [18], then Griesbach, Kennedy and Purves [19] found that hypophysectomy, removal of the pituitary gland, prevented occurrence of these goitres. This showed that these goitres were caused by thyroid-stimulating hormone from the pituitary, indicating that the brassica seed diets caused goitres by inhibiting thyroid hormone secretion. Kennedy climaxed these studies by showing that thioureas are goitrogenic and therefore could be used as medical treatment for thyrotoxicosis [20]. EB

Fig. 1.2 A Maori lady in the 1920s, with a goitre produced by iodine deficiency. An in vitro correlate of the Hayflick effect limits the mitotic capacity of unmutated thyroid cells in response to stimulation by the pituitary gland's thyroid-stimulating hormone [14]. Large goitres such as this are presumably due to somatic mutation of thyroid cells, comparable to "transformation" of a cell in tissue culture, i.e. this goitre is a benign tumour

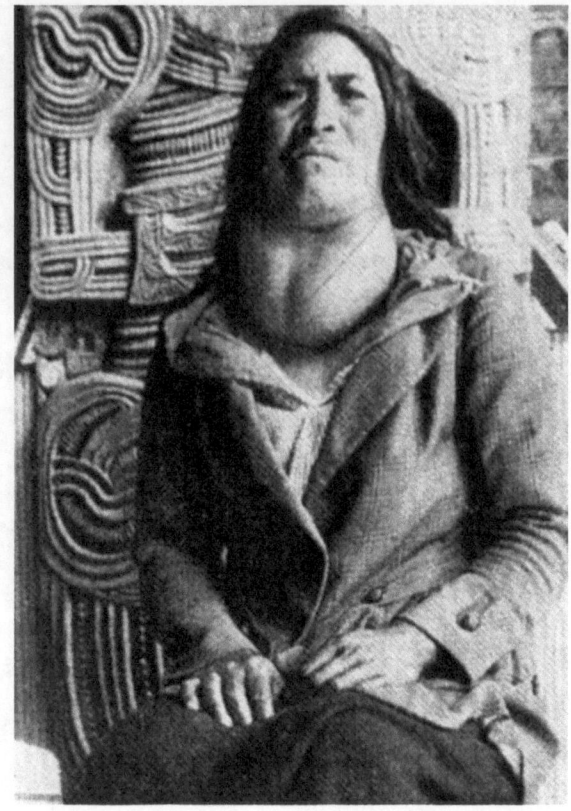

Astwood [21] later made the same discovery when exploring side effects of sulphonamides. Hence, a medical treatment for thyrotoxicosis became available, as an alternative to surgical subtotal thyroidectomy.

Solution of Pituitary Gland Cytology

The anterior pituitary gland is the conductor of the endocrine orchestra, relating the hypothalamus of the brain to the thyroid, adrenal, ovarian, mammary and testicular glands. With superb technology, relating cytological appearances to variety of functional states, Purves and Griesbach [22] identified the individual cells making thyrotrophin and the gonadotrophins, with a spectacular figure showing the spacial distribution of thyrotrophs and gonadotrophs in the pars distalis of the anterior pituitary gland. This research culminated in identification of all the hormone-secreting pituitary cells [23].

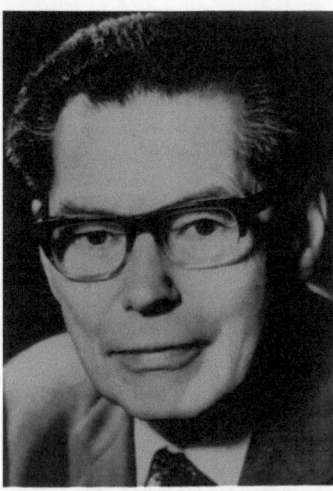

Fig. 1.3 Dr HD Purves. MSc, MB ChB, FRSNZ physicist, chemist, mathematician, clinician. With CE Hercus abolished NZ's goitre endemic, saving thyroid operations and birth of cretinous children. With TH Kennedy discovered antithyroid drugs, providing non-surgical treatment for thyrotoxicosis. With WE Griesbach solved pituitary cytology, finding which cell made which hormone. With DD Adams discovered the thyroid-stimulating autoantibodies that cause thyrotoxicosis

Adams' Entry into the Research World

As Professor of Public Health and Preventive Medicine at Otago Medical School, Charles Hercus followed classic academic practice in requiring his 5th year medical students to write a thesis, on any topic they chose, giving scope for originality. Adams, coming into Medicine to seek the cause of asthma, tested whether asthmatics make higher titres of antibodies to TAB vaccine than non-asthmatics. They do not, but Hercus marked Adams (Fig. 1.4) for future research and duly pulled him out of the MRACP stream of House Surgeon aspirants to work under HD Purves on the application of the newly available radioactive iodine to research on thyroid disease, in the MRC Endocrinology Research Unit. Signing a form for Adams' Research Fellowship, his very unusual clinical chief, Bill Fogg, Surgeon, Hospital Superintendent and previous professor of physiology, said,

"Even if you only stay with Purves one year, it will change you, it will make you think differently."

This astounded Adams, how could he think better than he did at present? Within two weeks under Purves' authority he understood. In ordinary clinical work, one has to make quick decisions, often on the basis of inadequate evidence. This is destructive of precise reasoning. In research, one is free to use strict logic, leaving decisions unmade until the evidence warrants it. This was a joy to Adams, the requirement to combine bold, fearless imagination with strict

Fig.1.4 Dr Duncan Adams, MD DSc FRACP. Selected by Dean Hercus for professional research, on the basis of a student thesis on asthma, Adams was apprenticed to HD Purves to use radioactive iodine in thyroid research. This led to discovery of the thyroid-stimulating autoantibodies that cause Graves' disease, confirmation of Burnet's Forbidden Clone Theory, and with JG Knight, The H Gene Theory, solution of the genetics of the autoimmune diseases

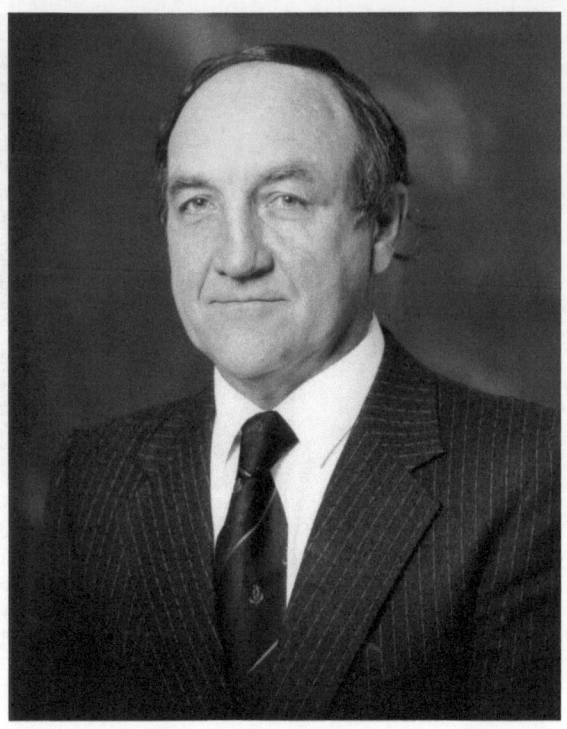

logical reasoning, all submitted to statistical measurement of probabilities, pioneered by R. A. Fisher, using Student's T test for significance of differences in magnitude of features and the Chi square test for significance of differences in the size of groups. For medical researchers, George Snedecor's "Statistical Methods" is a beautifully simple guide [24].

Graves' Disease

A thyroid disease, distinct from iodine-deficiency goitre, is Graves' disease, with thyroid enlargement, weight loss, staring eyes and a rapid pulse (Fig. 1.6). Out of the mass of incomprehensible diseases of the day, this clinical syndrome was recognised in 1835 by the Dublin physician, Robert Graves [25].

A century later, Sir Charles Harington [26] determined the atomic structure of the thyroid hormone, the first hormone to be so identified, finding it to be tetra-iodothyronine, containing four atoms of iodine. Harington named the thyroid hormone **thyroxine**. Its iodine content explained the role of iodine-deficiency in causation of goitre.

The cause of the thyroid gland overactivity of Graves' disease remained unknown, but was suspected to be a brain defect that caused excessive secretion of thyroid-stimulating hormone (TSH) by the pituitary gland.

Radioactive Iodine

Thanks to the atomic goldmine discovered by Baron Rutherford of Nelson [27], radioactive iodine became available for use in diagnosis, therapy and research into thyroid disease. Rutherford's use of a magnetic field to discover the α rays (positively charged, helium nuclei), β rays (negatively charged, electrons) and γ rays (uncharged) emitted by radium was a huge advance, and led to availability of radioactive elements for medical research. For thyroid research, radioactive iodine was the one needed. Ordinary iodine has an atomic weight of 127, but with an atomic weight of 131, radioactive iodine emits long-range γ rays, enabling measurements of iodine in the thyroids of people, and very short-range β rays (electrons) that destroy thyroid cells for therapy of Graves' disease, and are ideal for measurements of the radioactive iodine content of samples of blood.

Thyroid Research with Radioactive Iodine

Purves, a brilliant mathematician, chemist, physicist and clinician, provided his pupil, Adams, with superb tools for precise measurement of ^{131}I iodine in both people and laboratory animals, and in samples of their blood, housed in the new Hercus Building (Fig. 1.5). Dissatisfied with the development of technology for diagnosis and treatment of thyroid disease, Adams sought a more fundamental research project. There at hand was Graves' disease (Fig. 1.6), with unknown aetiology. It was not an infection, not a neoplasm, not present from birth, yet it ran in families. Compared to more common and less treatable diseases, Graves' disease was hardly of major importance, yet it seemed to Adams that discovery of its aetiology might reveal a fundamental new principle of disease and so was worth a major investment of time and effort. In 1951 the outstanding question was whether the thyroid hyper-secretion was caused by a nervous system defect mediated by hyper-secretion of thyroid-stimulating hormone (TSH) from the pituitary gland. The medical establishment of the day, including the great JH Means of Boston, believed this to be so, and RW Rawson had purported experimental evidence in support. Purves, a rock of intellectual independence, was sceptical. Visiting Boston on a Carnegie Travelling Fellowship, Purves attended a Means-Presided Staff Round at Massachusetts General Hospital. Asked to comment on a discussion on the cause of thyrotoxicosis, Purves stated that he did not believe it was excessive secretion of thyroid-stimulating hormone.

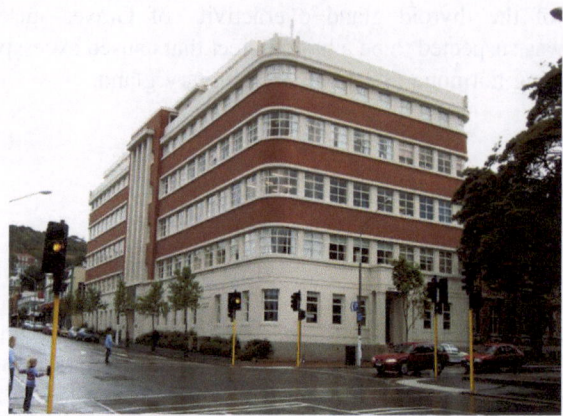

Fig. 1.5 The Hercus Building., *Fourth* floor Laboratory animals. *Third* floor Research units. *Second* floor Microbiology. *First* floor Pathology. *Ground* floor General practice. Intellectual "cross-fertilisation" by communication between floors

Fig. 1.6 A lady with Graves'disease, she has a diffusely enlarged thyroid, moderate exophthalmos with no defect of lid closure, she is euthyroid on methyl thiouracil and maintenance prednisone 10 mg/day for the exophthalmos [39]

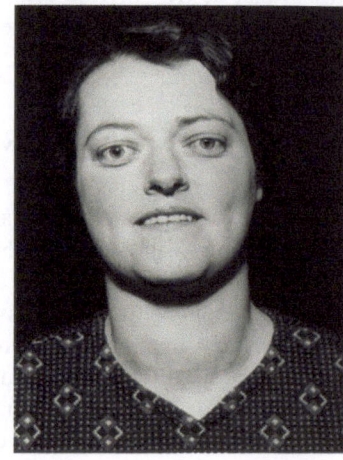

Means, "Tell us, Dr Purves, a single feature of Graves' disease not accounted for by an excess of thyroid-stimulating hormone!"

Purves' reply, "The lymphocytic infiltration!"

This shocked Means and galvanised the young doctors present.

Discovery of Long-Acting Thyroid Stimulator

In a proper interplay between wise, experienced teacher and energetic, ignorant pupil, Purves helped Adams develop a new TSH bioassay, aimed at determining whether blood TSH levels are raised in Graves' disease. After three years they had

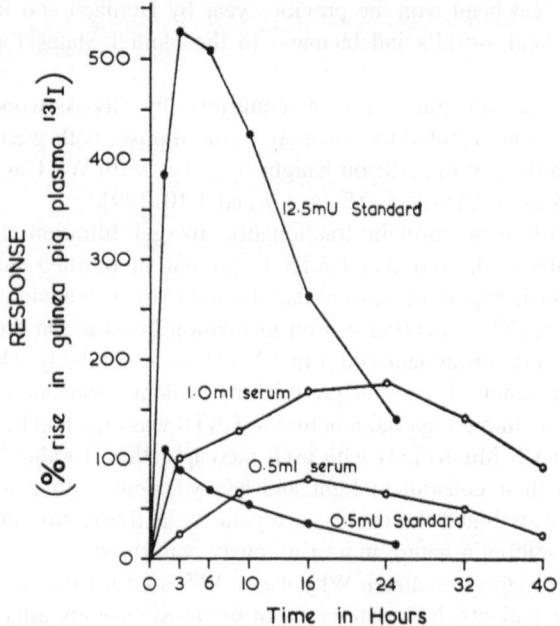

Fig. 1.7 The prolonged time course of the response elicited by two doses of serum from a case of thyrotoxicosis with exophthalmos (LATS) compared to two doses of USP standard TSH [9]

a guinea-pig assay that could readily measure the raised TSH levels in the blood of patients with the hypothyroid state, myxoedema. The principle was to inject the guinea pigs with ^{131}I as potassium iodide, thereby labelling their intra-thyroidal thyroid hormone. The secretion of this was inhibited by cold thyroxine injections, which acted by inhibiting the animals' secretion of pituitary TSH. After three days, the blood ^{131}I level reached a low steady level, but the thyroid was full of labelled thyroid hormone ready for release. Injections of TSH caused thyroid hormone secretion, raising the blood ^{131}I level. The magnitude of the response was remarkably sensitive to dosage of TSH, making the assay precise. As the animals did not need to be killed, Purves suggested using them repeatedly, so that variations in the sensitivity of individual animals could be determined. Hence the animals were used on three successive days. This proved to be a most fortunate step in revealing a long-acting substance. Serum from several Graves' patients had little effect, but Dr JA Kilpatrick's patient, Mrs McCabe, with exophthalmos, had something in her serum that had a prolonged effect, maximal 24 h after injection instead of the expected 3 h (Fig. 1.7), hence the name **long-acting thyroid stimulator (LATS)**.

With chemical expertise, Purves swiftly found LATS to be in the gamma globulins. This immediately raised the possibility that it was an antibody.

Finding LATS in other patients with Graves' disease, but not in all, Adams submitted an essay to the American Goiter Association, earning their Van Meter

Prize [9]. This had been won the previous year by Doniach and Roitt [7], illustrating the medical world's indebtedness to the United States for her research leadership.

The LATS phenomenon was soon confirmed by EB Astwood's pupil, JM McKenzie [28], who adapted the bioassay to the **mouse**, with great advantage.

Switching to the Mouse, Allison Knight (Fig. 1.8) with WS Cague and Adams steadily refined the LATS assay (Figs. 1.9 and 1.10) [29].

JP Kriss [30], using protein fractionation by gel filtration through DEAE Sephadex columns, showed that LATS is present in purified immunoglobulin preparations. Furthermore, he showed that thyroid extracts contain a molecule that will react with LATS to neutralise it on incubation in vitro. On the basis of this, Kriss made the first prominent claim that LATS is an antibody. He also showed that topical corticosteroids cure the pretibial myxoedema associated with very high LATS levels. The immunoglobulin nature of LATS was clinched by BR Smith, KJ Dorrington and DS Munro [31] who used mercaptoethanol reduction to split the molecules into their constituent light and heavy chains with loss of biological activity, then recombined the chains to regain the activity. No autoantibody has had its immunoglobulin nature more rigorously confirmed.

But a great mystery remained. Why was LATS absent from more than half of Graves' disease patients, including many of the most severely affected ones? The explanation soon came.

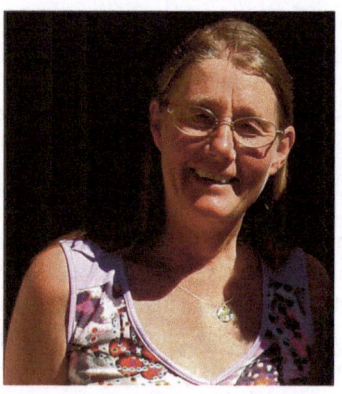

Fig. 1.8 Dr Allison Knight, BSc (Hons) PhD, With DDA showed that thyroid-stimulating autoantibodies show a fine variation between patients, in confirmation of the Forbidden Clone theory and that there is no allotypic variation in the autoantigen for the TSab [40]. In family studies, with Barbosa, showed that type1 diabetes is not caused by autoantibodies., Diabetes Research 1988; 9:1. It is now known to be caused by T cell autoimmunity. An opposite result in similar study of schizophrenic families would confirm a basis in B cell autoimmunity

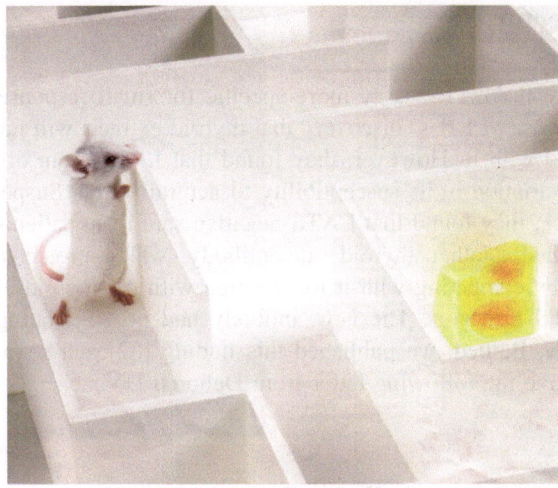

Fig. 1.9 A laboratory mouse in a maze, seeking a piece of cheese. Hundreds of mice were used to discover the features of the thyroid-stimulating autoantibodies. Because of the use of radioactive iodine these mice did not have to suffer, being bled from and injected into tail veins dilated by having the mice warm and not frightened. After each experiment they were euthanased with barbiturate

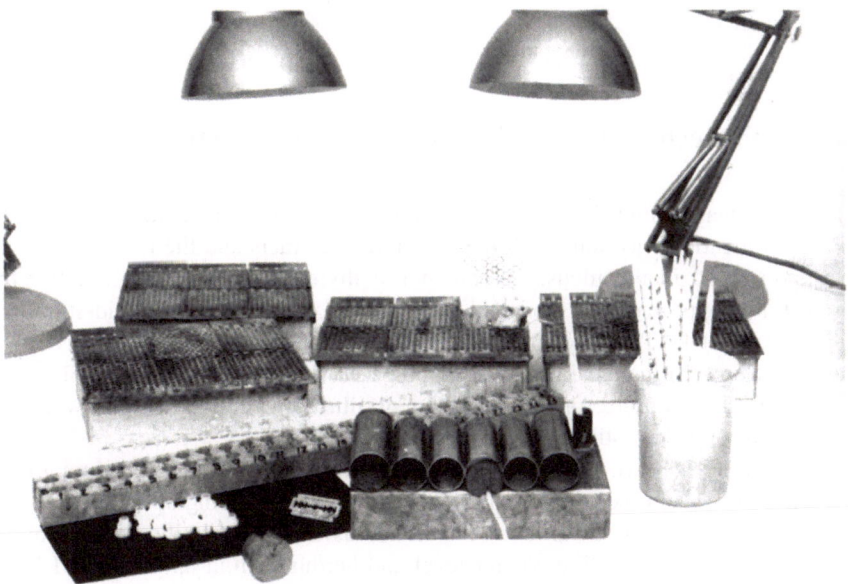

Fig. 1.10 Bioassay scene, including the mouse-warming apartments under overhead lamps, the mouse holder for tail vein bleeding by razor blade nick, and the pipettes for drawing up the blood for transfer into the vials in the wooden block

LATS Protector

Trying to make the LATS assay more specific for small responses, Adams and Kennedy made use of Kriss' discovery that thyroid extracts will neutralize LATS when incubated with it. However, they found that LATS from different patients showed wide variation in its susceptibility to neutralization. Suspecting an interfering substance, they found that LATS-negative sera from patients with Graves' disease contained another thyroid autoantibody, which protected LATS from neutralization by competing with it for reaction with the thyroid antigen. Hence, the name LATS protector. The new antibody had no stimulating effect in the mouse bioassay. Baffled, we published this finding [32] and soon had the good fortune to receive the following letter from Deborah Doniach.

A Letter from Deborah Doniach

London, May 5th, 1967.
    Dear Duncan,
    I wonder why you assume that the new LATS blocking antibody is not active in vivo? It could be more species specific and therefore not show up in the mouse test, yet still have stimulating properties on the human thyroid.
    Best wishes,
    Deborah Doniach.

LATS Protector, the Specific Human Thyroid Stimulator

Ivan Roitt was behind this brilliant interpretation, which was entirely logical, as the neutralization was done with human thyroid extracts and the test for activity was performed in the mouse. When mouse thyroid extracts were used LATS protector disappeared [33]. For final confirmation of the human thyroid-stimulating activity of LATS protector, it was necessary to round up half a dozen courageous Dunedin medical academics prepared to make themselves bioassay animals for LATS protector. This experiment, illustrated in Fig. 1.11, showed that LATS protector does stimulate the human thyroid [34].

With RDH Stewart and TH Kennedy, Adams showed LATS protector to be present in 90 % of cases of untreated Graves' disease including all the severe and moderately severe ones. Furthermore, there was a highly significant correlation between a patient's LATS protector level and her/his thyroid uptake of ^{131}I [35].

Figure 1.12 illustrates the pathogenesis of Graves' disease. It originates from a forbidden clone of lymphocytes, which would have developed into plasma cells, able to secrete large amounts of thyroid-stimulating autoantibodies (TSaab). These

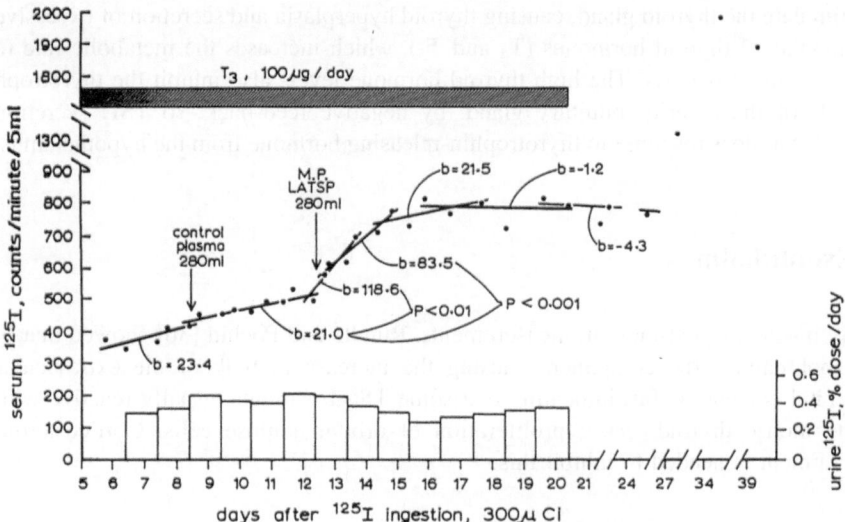

Fig. 1.11 The effect of infusion of LATS protector (LATSP) into a human volunteer. A control infusion of normal plasma has had no effect on the slowly rising blood ^{125}I level, but the LATSP infusion has caused a prominent and significant rise, indicating the occurrence of thyroid stimulation [34]

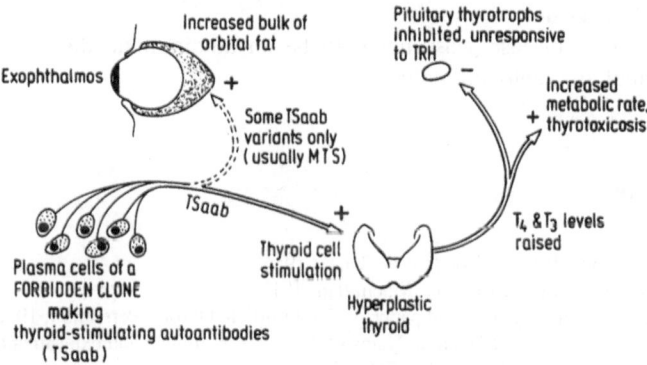

Fig. 1.12 The pathogenesis of Graves' disease. TSaab from forbidden clones of immunocytes stimulate the thyroid cells, causing overproduction of thyroid hormones T_4 and T_3 and the manifestations of thyrotoxicosis. The thyrotroph cells of the anterior pituitary are inhibited by the high blood thyroid hormone level, so TSH secretion ceases and response to TRH is absent. Some variants of TSaab react with receptors on fat cells in the orbit to cause exophthalmos from the bulk of adipocyte proliferation, demonstrated by Rundle and Pochin [10, 36]

stimulate the thyroid gland, causing thyroid hyperplasia and secretion of excessive amounts of thyroid hormones (T_4 and T_3), which increases the metabolic rate to cause thyrotoxicosis. The high thyroid hormone levels also inhibit the thyrotroph cells of the anterior pituitary gland, by negative feed-back, so TSH secretion ceases as does response to thyrotrophin-releasing hormone from the hypothalamus.

Exophthalmos

By ingenious post-mortem measurements, Rundle and Pochin [36] showed that in exophthalmos the component causing the increase in bulk of the extra-ocular orbital contents is **fat,** indicating that some TSaab variants, usually reactive with the mouse thyroid, cause proliferation of orbital adipose cells. Corticosteroid treatment is needed to inhibit this.

Neonatal Thyrotoxicosis

A quintessence of precision in the measurement of a pathogenic autoantibody was achieved by SM Dirmikis, DS Munro et al. [37] who defined units of LATS protector, then showed that maternal LATS protector levels over 20 units/ml invariably give rise to neonatal thyrotoxicosis in babies, whereas levels below 10 units/ml never do.

Thus Graves' disease was shown to be an autoimmune disease, caused by thyroid-stimulating autoantibodies [38].

References

1. Dubos RJ. Louis Pasteur. London: Gallancz; 1956.
2. Godlee RJ. Lord Lister. London: Macmillan; 1917.
3. Himmelweit F. ed. The collected papers of Paul Ehrlich. Oxford: Pergamon; 1956. p. 205–12.
4. Dameshek W, Schwartz SO. Hemolysins as the cause of clinical and experimental hemolytic anemias. Am J Med Sci. 1938;196:769–92.
5. Witebsky E, Rose N, Terplan K, Paine JR, Egan RW. Chronic thyroiditis and autoimmunization. JAMA. 1957;164:1439–47.
6. Freund J, Lipton MM, Thompson GE. Aspermatogenesis in the guinea pig induced by testicular tissue and adjuvants. J Exp Med. 1953;97:711.
7. Doniach D, Roitt IM. Autoimmunity in Hashimoto's disease and its implications. J Clin Endocrinol Metab. 1957;17:1293–304.
8. Adams DD, Purves HD. Abnormal responses in the assay of thyrotrophin. Proc Univ Otago Med Sch. 1956;34:11–2.
9. Adams DD. The presence of an abnormal thyroid-stimulating hormone in the serum of some thyrotoxic patients. J Clin Endocrinol Metab. 1958;18:699–712.

10. Adams DD. Thyroid-stimulating autoantibodies. Vitam Horm. 1980;38:119–203.
11. Coombs RRA, Gell PGH. The classification of allergic reactions underlying disease. In: Coombs RRA, Gell PGH, editors. Clinical aspects of immunology. Philadelphia: Davis; 1962. p. 319.
12. Johnson KJ, Chensue SW, Kunkel SL, Ward PA. Immunologically mediated tissue injury. In: Rubin E, FaberJ, editors. Pathology, 2nd edn, Philadelphia: Lippincott; 1994. p. l05–17.
13. Adams DD, Knight JG. Principles of autoimmune disease: pathogenesis genetics and specific immunotherapy. J Clin Lab Immunol. 2003; 52:1–22.
14. Hercus CE, Benson WN, Carter CL. Endemic goitre in New Zealand and its relation to the soil iodine. J Hyg. 1925;24:321–402.
15. Kelly EC, Snedden WW. Prevalence and geographical distribution of endemic goitre. Geneva: World Health Organization, Palais des Nations; 1960.
16. Purves Symposium. New Zealand Med J. 1974–5; 80–81: 475, 548, 15, 61.
17. Chesney AM, Clawson T A, Webster B. Johns Hopkins Hosp Bull 1928; 43:261.
18. Kennedy TH, Purves HD. Studies on experimental goitre. 1: The effect of brassica seed diets on rats. Brit J Exp Path. 1941; 22:241–4.
19. Griesbach WE, Kennedy TH, Purves HD. Studies on experimental goitre. III: the effect of goitrogenic diet on hypophysectomized rats. Brit J Exp Path. 1941; 22:249–51.
20. Kennedy TH. Thioureas as goitrogenic substances. Nature. 1942;150:233–4.
21. Astwood EB. Treatment of hyperthyroidism with thiourea and thiouracil. JAMA. 1943;251:1743–6.
22. Purves HD, Griesbach WE. The site of thyrotrophin and gonadotrophin production in the rat pituitary studied by McManus-Hotchkiss staining for glycoprotein. Endocrinology. 1951;49:244–64.
23. Purves HD. Cytology of the adenohypophysis. In: Harris GW, Donovan BT, editors. The pituitary gland. London: Butterworths; 1966. p. 147–232.
24. Snedecor GW. Statistical methods. 5th ed. Ames: Iowa StateUniversity Press; 1956.
25. Graves RJ. Clinical lectures. London Med Surg J. 1835;7:513.
26. Harington CR. The thyroid gland. London: Oxford University Press; 1933.
27. Gribbin, J. Science. A history 1543–2001. London: Penguin Books; 2003. p. 499–506.
28. McKenzie JM. Delayed thyroid response to serum from thyrotoxic patients. Endocrinology. 1958;62:865–8.
29. Knight A, Cague WS, Adams DD. Measurements of thyroid-stimulating autoantibodies. In: Rose NR, Friedman H. editors. Manual of clinical immunology. 2nd ed. Washington: American Society for Microbiology; 1980. p. 391–402.
30. Kriss JP, Pleshakov V, Chien JR. Isolation and identification of the long-acting thyroid stimulator and its relation to hyperthyroidism and circumscribed pretibial myxoedema. J Clin Endocrinol Metab. 1964;24:1005–28.
31. Smith BR, Dorrington KJ, Munro DS. The thyroid-stimulating properties of long-acting thyroid stimulator and γ-globulin subunits. Biochem Biophys Acta. 1969;192:277–85.
32. Adams DD, Kennedy TH. Occurrence in thyrotoxicosis of a gamma globulin which protects LATS from neutralization by an extract of thyroid gland. J Clin Endocrinol Metab. 1967;27:173–7.
33. Adams DD, Kennedy TH. Evidence to suggest that LATS-P stimulates the human thyroid gland. J Clin Endocrinol Metab. 1971;33:47–51.
34. Adams DD, Fastier FN, Howie JB, Kennedy TH, Kilpatrick JA, Stewart RDH. Stimulation of the human thyroid by infusions of plasma containing LATS protector. J Clin Endocrinol Metab. 1974;39:826–32.
35. Adams DD, Kennedy TH, Stewart RDH. Correlation between long-acting thyroid stimulator protector level and thyroid ^{131}I uptake in thyrotoxicosis. Brit Med J. 1974;2:199–201.
36. Rundle F, Pochin E. The orbital tissues in thyrotoxicosis: a quantitative analysis relating to exophthalmos. Clin Sci. 1944;5:51–74.

37. Munro DS, Dirmikis SM, Humphries H, Smith T, Broadhead GD. The role of thyroid-stimulating immunoglobulins of Graves' disease in neonatal thyrotoxicosis. Brit J Obst Gyn. 1978;85:837–43.
38. Adams DD, Knight A, Knight JG, Laing P. Graves' disease; a paradigm for autoimmunity. In: Pinchera A, Ingbar SH, McKenzie JM, Fenzi GF. editors. Thyroid autoimmun. New York: Plenum; 1987. p. 1–10.
39. Adams DD. Long-acting thyroid stimulator: how receptor autoimmunity was discovered. Autoimmunity. 1988;1:3–9.
40. Knight A, Cague WS, Adams DD. Measurement of the thyroid-stimulating autoantibodies. In: Rose NR, Friedman H, editors. Manual of clinical immunology. 2nd ed. Washington: American Society for Microbiology; 1980. p. 391–402.
41. Jarrett EE, Miller HR. Production and activities of IgE in helminth infection. Prog Allergy. 1982;31:178–233.
42. Bell RG. IgE, allergies and helminth parasites; a new perspective on an oldconundrum. Immunol Cell Biol. 1996;74:337–45.
43. Adams DD. Autoimmune mechanisms. In: Davies TF, editor. Autoimmune endocrine disease. New York: Wiley; 1983. p. 1–39.
44. Adams DD. Systemic lupus erythaematosus: a simple concept of the pathogenesis and its genetic basis. In: Dawkins RL, Christiansen FT, Zilko PJ, editors. Immunogenetics in rheumatology. Amsterdam: Excerpta Medica; 1982. p. 242–3.
45. Lindstrom J, Shelton D, Fujii Y. Myasthenia gravis. Adv Immunol. 1988;42:233–84.
46. Ebringer A, Rashid T, Wilson C. Rheumatoid arthritis, *Proteus,* anti-CCP antibodies and Karl Popper. Autoimmune Rev. 2010;9:216–23.
47. Sherwin RS. Diabetes mellitus. In: Goldman L, Bennett JC, editors. Cecil textbook of medicine 21st edn. Philadelphia: Saunders; 2000. P. 1263–85.
48. Sutherland DE, Goetz FC, Sibley RE. Recurrence of disease in pancreas transplants. Diabetes. 1989;38:85.
49. Klintworth GK. The eye. In: Rubin E, Farber JL, editors. Pathology. 2nd ed. Philadelphia: Lippincott; 1988. p. 1456–83.
50. Adams DD. Autoimmune destruction of pericytes as the cause of diabetic retinopathy. Clin Ophthalmol. 2008;2:295–8.
51. Ben-Nun A, Wekerle H, Cohen I. The rapid isolation of clonable antigenic-specific T cell lines capable of mediating autoimmune encephalomyelitis. Eu J Immunol. 1981;11:195–9.

Chapter 2
Pathogenesis

Immune Tolerance

In World War II, British fighter pilots defending England from bombing by the Nazi Luftwaffe, sometimes survived with terrible burns to the face and hands. This caused surgeons to attempt to heal them with skin grafts and led Medawar to study the fate of grafts performed between rabbits [1]. He found that second set grafts were rejected faster than first set ones, in conformity with immune system mediation of the graft rejection. Becoming interested in preventing allograft rejection by artificial induction of immune tolerance, non-reactivity to specific antigens, Medawar and his colleagues inoculated new-born mice with specific cells and showed that sometimes this produced non-reactivity when the animals had become adult [2]. This led to the idea that in animals, around the time of birth, there is a **D day**, when the immunity system changes from permanent non-reactivity (tolerance) to antigens, which will be host ones, to reactivity to new antigens, which will be foreign ones on invading microbes.

Nossal's Key Experiment

In a beautiful experiment, shown in Fig. 2.1, Nossal and Pike [3], culturing bone marrow cells from adult animals, showed that **D day, for change from tolerance to an antigen to immune reactivity against it,** is not a stage in the life of an animal, but a stage in the life of every new lymphocyte clone. This enables the histocompatibility antigens, major, minor and HY (the male histocompatibility antigen), always present where lymphocytes are multiplying, to police the immune repertoire by deleting any new B or T lymphocyte clone with a complementary antigen receptor [4]. By natural selection of reproductive advantage, sets of **immune response genes**, coding for histocompatibility antigens and antigen receptors on B and T lymphocytes, have evolved, over many generations, to maximise defence against current microbial diseases and to minimise autoimmune disease [5].

D. D. Adams and C. D. Adams, *Autoimmune Disease,*
SpringerBriefs in Public Health, DOI: 10.1007/978-94-007-6937-3_2,
© The Author(s) 2013

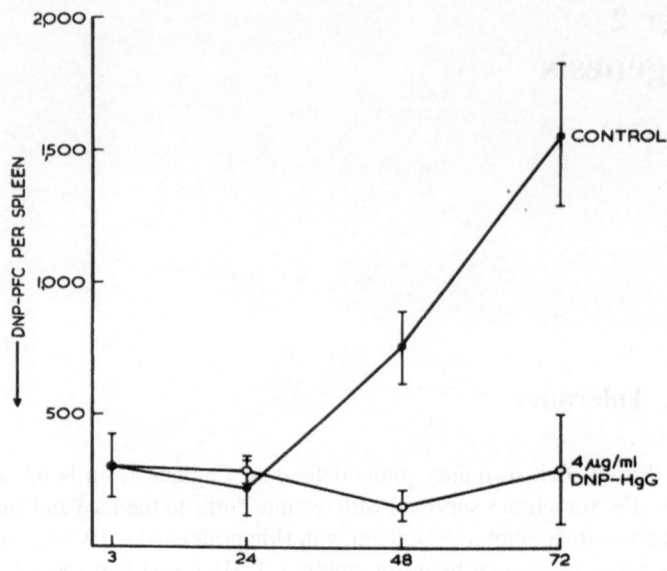

Fig. 2.1 Evidence for clonal abortion by antigenic contact in immature bone marrow lymphocytes from adult mice. These cells differentiate during 72 h in culture, to acquire antibody-secreting capacity (curve labelled "control") as shown by the plaque-forming cell (PFC) technique. If an antigen (in the experiment illustrated, dinitrophenol on human gamma globulin, DNP-HgG) is present in the medium, reactivity to it does not develop (curve labelled 4 µg/ml DNP-HgG). This experiment shows that D day for the switch from tolerance to immune reaction is not a stage in the life of an animal, but a stage in the life of every new lymphocyte clone, arising by the frequent somatic mutations in the V genes of multiplying lymphocytes [3]

Discovery of the Structure of Antibody Molecules

Serum, which is blood from which red cells and white cells have been removed, contains dissolved proteins, including the gamma globulins that are now called immunoglobulins because they are the antibodies. How could the atomic structure of such a great mixture of molecules be determined? Henry Kunkel solved this problem by using blood from patients with multiple myeloma, a cancer in which a lymphocyte cell becomes malignant, producing large amounts of a single antibody molecule. Kunkel's pupil, Gerald Edelman, broke the disulphide bonds holding antibodies together, revealing that each antibody molecule is comprised of four amino acid chains, two long ones and two short ones, the disulphide bonds holding them together to form a functional antibody. Rodney Porter [6] successfully split antibody molecules into their constituent amino acid chains, by using the weak proteolytic enzyme, papain. This produced three fragments, a Crystallizable Fragment, FC, the constant region, and two identical Fragments, FAB, each of which formed identical Antigen Binding sites. Figure 2.2 shows this structure.

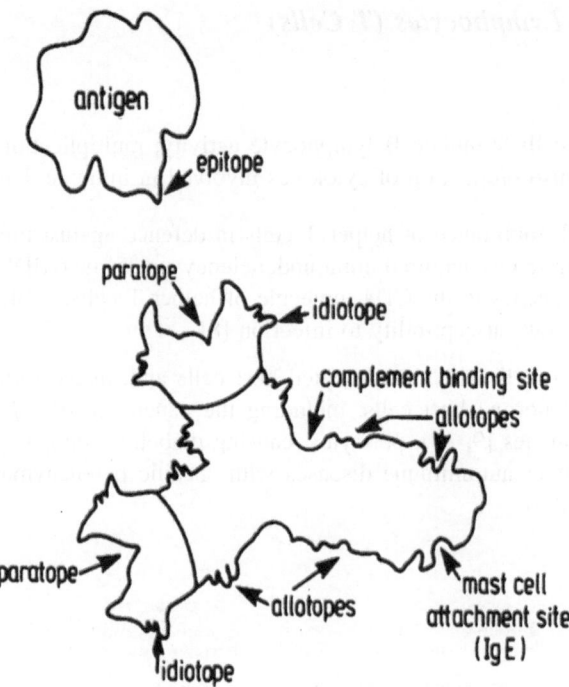

Fig. 2.2 An antibody molecule of IgG class showing the two identical *paratopes* (combining sites for antigen) and the complimentary *epitope* of the antigen molecule. Also shown are the *idiotopes* (constant region epitopes) and the attachment sites for the C1q molecule of the complement system. Additionally, an attachment site for mast cells present on IgE class antibody molecules is depicted [4]

Discovery of T and B Lymphocytes

Some years after Haldane had discovered the histocompatibility system, as described below in **Genetics**, his nephew, Mitchison [7], in a classical experiment, showed that rejection of allografts is not mediated by antibodies, but that lymphocyte cells are necessary, the rejection therefore being appropriately described as "cell-mediated." This was the discovery of the **cytotoxic T lymphocytes** that bear the CD8 (cluster of differentiation antigens 8) surface marker and are essential for defence against virus infection. Mitchison also discovered the **helper T lymphocytes** that bear the CD4 surface marker and are necessary for firing off the cytokine secretions that mediate the cell cooperation involved in an immune attack on an invading microbe. The lymphocytes which act by secreting antibodies became known as **B lymphocytes**, because of their origin from the bone marrow, whereas **T lymphocytes** are named for their origin in the thymus.

Types of T Lymphocytes (T Cells)

There are three.

1. **Helper T cells** stimulate B lymphocyte activity, multiplication and antibody secretion, also production of cytokines involved in immune defence.

   The crucial importance of helper T cells in defence against infection is strikingly demonstrated by acquired immunodeficiency syndrome (AIDS), in which the HIV-1 virus attaches to the CD4 molecule of helper T cells, depleting them and causing dangerous susceptibility to infection [8]

2. **Cytotoxic T cells** kill virus-infected host cells and, in the form of forbidden clones, kill normal host cells, including the pancreatic islet β cells, causing Type 1 Diabetes [9, 10], pericytes, causing diabetic retinopathy [11, 12] and probably other autoimmune diseases with specific parenchymal cell destruction. (Fig. 2.3)

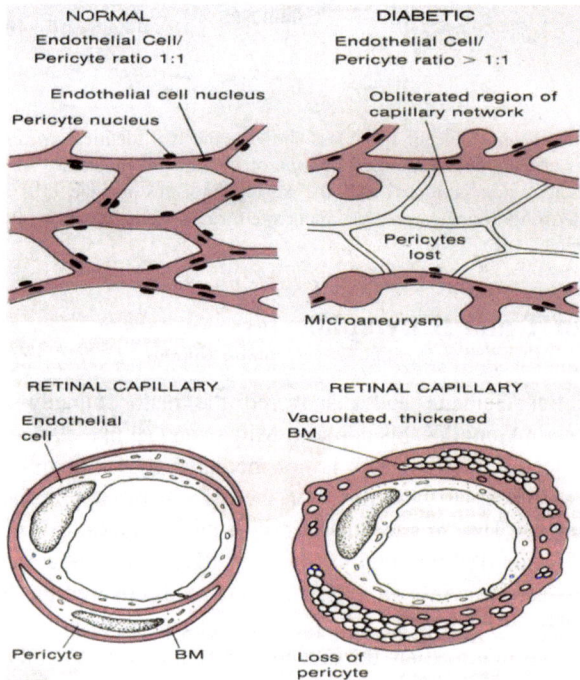

Fig. 2.3 Association of pericyte loss with collapse of the retinal vasculature in diabetic retinopathy., Adams has postulated that the pericytes are destroyed by forbidden clones of cytotoxic T cells, antigenicly-related to those that destroy the pancreatic islet β cells. So therapy should be immunosuppression, not ineffective strict glycaemic control. (Clin Ophthalmol 2008; 2:295–8.). From [12]

3. **Suppressor T** cells inhibit immune reactions.

This was discovered in Japan by Sakaguchi and colleagues [13], who found that neonatal thymectomy caused autoimmune destruction of ovaries in mice, and in Scotland, where Irvine and colleagues [14] found that autoimmune thyroiditis in T cell-depleted rats could be suppressed by normal lymphocytes.

After development of **monoclonal antibody technology** had enabled discovery of the many clusters of differentiation (CD) antigens on lymphocytes [15], the CD4 cluster were found on helper T lymphocytes and the CD8 cluster on cytotoxic lymphocytes that destroy virus-infected cells. The CD25 cluster was found on suppressor T cells and to be part of the cell's receptor for the cytokine, interleukin-2 (Il-2), which was originally known as **T cell growth factor**, because it enabled T cells to be grown in vitro.

Regulation of Immune Responses

Natchtigal, Zan-Bar and Feldman [16] provide an explanation for the mechanism by which T cells regulate immune responses, as shown in Fig. 2.4. They postulate that

1. **Immature T cells**, meeting complementary antigen, differentiate into suppressor T cells, which suppress the specific immune response.
2. **Mature T cells**, become helper T cells.

This regulatory function of T cells effectively controls the magnitude of an immune response, preventing it continuing on indefinitely until somatic mutations

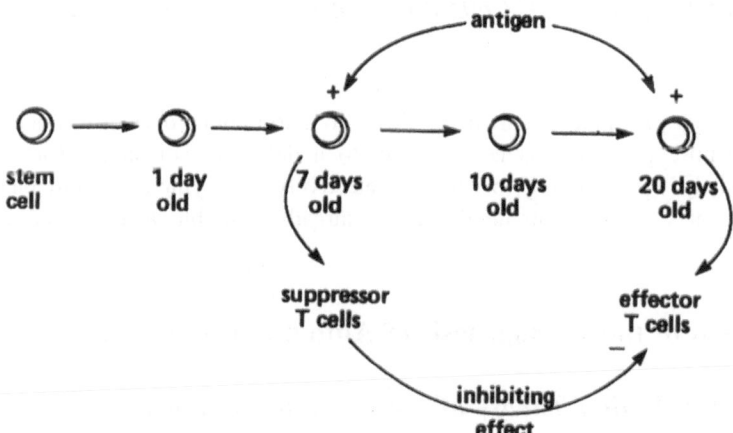

Fig. 2.4 The hypothesis of Natchtigal et al. [13]; immature T cells, meeting complementary antigen differentiate into suppressor T cells, in contrast to mature T cells which become effector T cells. This mechanism effectively controls the magnitude of an immune response, inhibiting both leukaemia and autoimmunity [16]

in the multiplying lymphocytes lead to leukaemia or autoimmune disease. Hence, suppressor T cells are a vital element of the functioning of the immune system [4].

Suppressor T Cells as the Cause of the Autoimmune Diseases

Allison, Denman and Barnes [17] postulated that loss of suppressor T cells is the cause of the autoimmune diseases. This was a very popular idea, but key purported evidence for the concept, repeated by Knight and Adams with larger numbers of mice and adequate statistics proved that the effect was not there [18].

In 1995, Sakaguchi [19], using lymphocyte cell-sorting technology and transfer of cells into lymphocyte-deficient mice, made the seminal observation that animals deprived of CD25+ lymphocytes develop autoimmune disease. After showing the existence of CD4+ CD25+ suppressor T cells in man, Shevach [20] reflected on their enormous potential for therapeutic use, but noted that no way of achieving this had been devised.

The gene, FOXP3, a transcriptional repressor that inhibits activation-induced Il-2 gene translation, has been shown to be both necessary and sufficient for the development and function of naturally arising CD4+ CD25+ suppressor T cells [21]. Children with defects of the FOXP3 gene die of immune-dysregulation, polyendocrinopathy, enteropathy, X-linked syndrome (IPEX) [22]. Furthermore, animals depleted of FOXP3+ lymphocytes, die of autoimmune disease.

In the last few years, efforts to use suppressor T cells for treatment of auto-immune diseases, or allograft rejection, or to remove them to enhance attack on tumours, have all been unsuccessful [23].

Loss of Suppressor T Cells does not Cause the Autoimmune Diseases

As Shevach [24] notes, apart from IPEX, no autoimmune disease has been iden-tified whose pathogenesis is secondary to a deficiency of suppressor T cells. Fortunately, the technology needed for selectively destroying the forbidden clones that do cause the autoimmune diseases is already available, as described below.

Solution of the Pathogenesis of Autoimmune Disease

Jerne's Selection Theory of the Immune Response

Because antibodies were known to fit their antigens closely, it was reasonable to think that they were built around the antigen, an idea that was expressed by

Horowitz as the template theory. However, after Watson and Crick's epochal solution [25] of the structure and function of DNA, Jerne [26] had the crucial realisation that cells' easy DNA to RNA to polypeptide manufacturing capacity, meant that antibodies could be pre-formed, in myriad diversity, awaiting contact with an antigen that fitted, like ready-made shoes in a shop awaiting a customer with the right-sized foot.

The Immunological Clone

If a potato is divided into pieces and these are put in the ground, the resultant group of genetically identical plants is known in horticulture as a "clone". Burnet [27] introduced this term to immunology to describe a group of immunocytes with identical receptors for antigen. Implicit in the clonal concept are two assumptions, namely;

(1) That a single immunocyte produces antibody of only one specificity and
(2) That antibody of a single specificity is produced by more than one immunocyte. Both these fundamentally important assumptions now have experimental confirmation.

Burnet's Clonal Selection Theory of the Immune Response

Building on Jerne's selection theory, Burnet realised that it is not antibodies that are selected, but the cells that make them, and that these are the **lymphocytes**. Furthermore, he realised that lymphocytes exist as clones of cells with identical receptors for antigen, there being millions of cells in each clone and millions of clones in a person. This is the Clonal Selection Theory of acquired immunity [27], today in general acceptance and illustrated in Fig. 2.5.

Burnet's Forbidden Clone Theory of Autoimmune Disease

As a bacteriologist, Burnet had counted mutation rates in populations of bacteria multiplying on blood agar plates. He realised that mutations would occur similarly in populations of multiplying lymphocytes. Coining the apt term "forbidden clone," for lymphocyte clones that react with a host antigen, Burnet postulated that these arise by somatic gene mutations in multiplying lymphocytes and are the cause of the autoimmune diseases [28]. This was confirmed for Graves' disease by demonstration that in individual patients, the thyroid-stimulating autoantibodies contain only one of two possible immunoglobulin light chain types, λ or κ, but

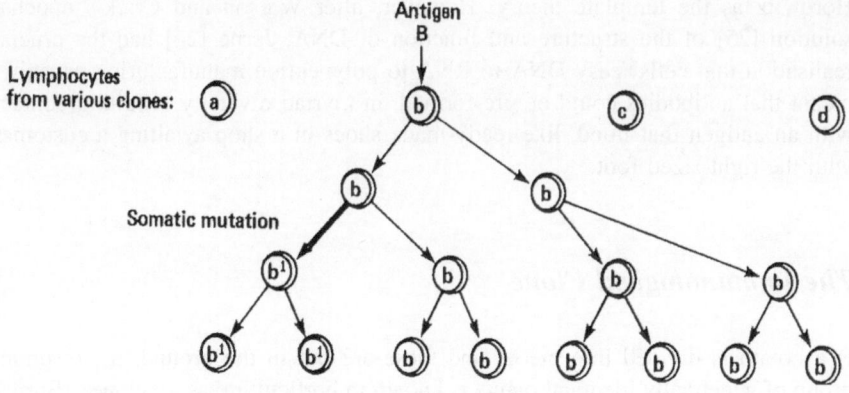

Fig. 2.5 Clonal selection by antigenic stimulation and clonal diversification by somatic mutation. Concept of Jerne [26] and Burnet [27] (Adams [4])

never both, and therefore arise from a single lymphocyte by somatic mutation in its V genes [29].

Cytotoxic T Cell Forbidden Clones

Sherwin's epic research on diabetes [9] has been capped by the discovery that the exquisitely-specific destruction of the pancreatic islet β cells that causes **Type 1 Diabetes** is caused by cytotoxic T cells [10]. Following this up, Adams has postulated that antigen receptor-related cytotoxic T cells destroy the retinal pericytes, which Klintworth [11] has shown to occur in **diabetic retinopathy** and that this is the cause of the vascular collapse of diabetic retinopathy [12] (Fig. 2.3). This indicates the need for replacement of tight glycaemic control as treatment for diabetic retinopathy by trial of immunosuppression.

Graves' Disease, a Paradigm for Autoimmune Disease

In 1986, at the University of Pisa, Professor Aldo Pinchera initiated and led an International Symposium on Thyroid Autoimmunity [30].

This was a culmination of understanding of the pathogenesis and genetics of autoimmune disease. Of all the autoimmune diseases, those involving the thyroid gland had unique advantages for study because of the presence of iodine in thyroid hormone, the hormone receptor nature of the Graves' disease autoantigen and the control of thyroid activity by the pituitary gland. Clear evidence, from world wide research supported the Forbidden Clone theory of the pathogenesis, and the H Gene theory of the genetics, described below [31].

Table 2.1 Discovered pathogenic forbidden clones and others awaiting discovery

Disease or disorder	Autoantigen	Cell type of the forbidden clone
Graves' disease	TSH receptor [34]	B cell, plasma cell
Myasthenia Gravis	Acetylcholine receptor [35]	"
Goodpasture's disease	On glomerular and lung basement membrane[36]	"
Pernicious anaemia	Intrinsic factor [37]	"
Systemic lupus erythaematosus	An intracellular component made copiously available by cytolysis [38]	"
"Thrombosis by lupus anticoagulant [40]	Platelet cell wall phospholipid [39]	"
Hypocomplementaemia	Alternative pathway C3 convertase abnormally stabilised by C3 nephritic factor [41]	"
Haemolytic anaemia	Red cell surface component [42]	"
Thrombocytopenia	Platelet surface component [43]	"
Rheumatoid arthritis	Type X1 collagen [44, 45]	"
Schizophrenia	A neuronal dopaminergic receptor [46, 47]	"
Manic depressive	?Another neuronal receptor	"
Systemic scleroderma	?Fibroblast receptor causing excessive collagen formation [48– 50]	"
Paget's disease	?Osteoclast receptor, causing bone resorption [51]	"
Post-streptococcal glomerulonephritis	?Intra-cellular glomerular component exposed by nephritogenic strep toxin	?B cell, as Ig is in the lesion [52]
Rheumatic fever	Heart component cross-reactive with streptococci [53]	?T cell as the heart autoantibodies also occur in uncomplicated strep infection [54]
Diabetes type 1	Islet β cell surface component	Cytotoxic CD8 T cell [9, 10]
Diabetic retinopathy	?Vascular pericyte cells	Cytotoxic T cell, CD8 [11, 12]
Autoimmune hepatitis	?Hepatocyte surface component	?Cytotoxic T cell, CD8 [55]
Addison's disease	?Adrenocortical cell surface component	?Cytotoxic T cell [56]
Primary biliary cirrhosis	?Ductal cell surface component[57]	?Cytotoxic T cell, CD8
Multiple sclerosis	?Oligodendrocyte surface component	?Cytotoxic T cell, CD8 [58]
Polymyositis	?Muscle cell surface component	CD8 α/β T cell [59]

Pathogenic Forbidden Clones; Discovered Ones and Ones Awaiting Discovery

These are shown in Table 2.1. Initially, discovery of forbidden clones depended on particular expertise in various non-immunological fields, such as endocrinology, with radioactive iodine for Graves' disease and neurology, with acetylcholine receptors from the electric eel and bungarotoxin from poisonous India arrows, for myasthenia gravis.

A promising way to seek new forbidden clones is to use the receptor-ligand technology invented by GP Smith [32, 33]. Patients' serum or cerebrospinal fluid can be screened on bacteriophage peptide display libraries to seek antibodies that are confined to certain autoimmune diseases. The blood–brain barrier may result in clones proliferating on the brain side of the barrier without significant representation on the blood side, where the stimulating antigen may not exist. Hence for seeking autoantibodies causing psychoses, cerebrospinal fluid may need to be the starting material.

References

1. Medawar PB. The behaviour and fate of skin autografts and skin homografts in rabbits. J Anat. 1944;78:176–99.
2. Billingham RE, Brent L, Medawar PB. Actively acquired tolerance of foreign cells. Nature. 1953;172:603–6.
3. Nossal JG, Pike B. Evidence for the clonal abortion theory of B lymphocyte tolerance. J Exp Med. 1975;141:904–17.
4. Adams DD. Autoimmune mechanisms. In: Davies TF, editor. Autoimmune endocrine disease. New York: Wiley; 1983. p. 1–39.
5. Adams DD, Knight JG. Principles of autoimmune disease: pathogenesis, genetics and specific immunotherapy. J Clin Lab Immunol. 2003;52:1–22.
6. Porter RR. The hydrolysis of rabbit globulin and antibodies with crystalline papain. Biochem J. 1959;73:119.
7. Mitchison NA. Passive transfer of transplantation immunity. Proc Roy Soc B. 1954;143:72–87.
8. Shaw GM. Biology of human immunodeficiency viruses. In: Goldman L, Bennett JC, editors. Textbook of medicine. 21st edn. Philadelphia: Saunders; 2000. p. 1893–8.
9. Sherwin RS. Diabetes mellitus. In: Goldman L, Bennett JC, editors. Cecil textbook of medicine. 21st edn. Philadelphia: Saunders; 2000. p. 1263–85.
10. Sutherland DE, Goetz FC, Sibley RE. Recurrence of disease in pancreas transplants. Diabetes. 1989;38:85.
11. Klintworth GK. The eye. In: Rubin E, Farber JL, editors. Pathology. 2nd ed. Philadelphia: Lippincott; 1988. p. 1456–83.
12. Adams DD. Autoimmune destruction of pericytes as the cause of diabetic retinopathy. Clin Ophthalmol. 2008;2:295–8.
13. Sakaguchi S, Takahashi T, Nishizuka Y. Study on cellular events in post-thymectomy autoimmune oophoritis in mice. II. Replacement of Lyt-1 cells in normal female mice for the prevention of oophoritis. J Exp Med. 1982;156:1577–86.

14. Penhale WJ, Irvine WJ, Inglis JR, Farmer A. Thyroiditis in T cell-depleted rats: suppression of the autoallergic response by re-constitution with normal lymphoid cells. Clin Exp Immunol. 1976;25:6–16.

15. Paul WE editor. Fundamental immunology. 4th edn. Philadelphia: Lippincott-Raven; 1999. p. 605–650.

16. Natchtigal D, Zan-Bar I, Feldman N. The role of specific suppressor T cells in immune tolerance. Transplant Rev. 1975;26:87–105.

17. Allison AC, Denman AM, Barnes AD. Hypothesis. Cooperating and controlling functions of thymus-derived lymphocytes in relation to autoimmunity. Lancet. 1971;2:135–40.

18. Knight JG, Adams DD. Failure of transferred thymus cells to suppress or prevent autoantibody production in NZB and NZB × NZW mice. J Clin Lab Immunol. 1978;1:151–8.

19. Sakaguchi S, Sakaguchi N, Asano M, Itoh M, Toda M. Immunologic self-tolerance maintained by activated T cells expressing IL-2 receptor α-chains (CD25). Breakdown of a single mechanism of self-tolerance causes various autoimmune diseases. J Immunol. 1995;160:1151–64.

20. Shevack EM. Certified professionals: CD4$^+$CD25$^+$ suppressor T cells. J Exp Med. 2001;193:41–6.

21. Lopes JE, Torgerson TR, Schubert LA, Anover SD, Ocheltree EL, Ochs HD, Ziegler SF. Analysis of FOXP3 reveals multiple domains required for its function as a transcriptional repressor. J Immunol. 2006;177:3133–42.

22. Bennett CL, Christie J, Ramsdell F, et al. The immune dysregulation, polyendocrinopathy, enteropathy, X-linked syndrome (IPEX) is caused by mutation of FOXP3. Nat Genet. 2001;7:20–1.

23. Sakaguchi S. Naturally-arising CD4+ regulatory T cells for immunologic self-tolerance and negative control of immune responses. Annu Rev Immunol. 2004;22:531–62.

24. Shevach EM. Organ-specfic autoimmunity. In: Paul WE, editor. Fundamental immunology. 4th edn. Philadelphia: Lippincott-Raven; 1999. p. 1089–125.

25. Watson JD, Crick FH. Molecular structure of nucleic acids. Nature. 1953;171:737–8.

26. Jerne NK. The natural selection theory of antibody formation. Proc Nat Acad Sci USA. 1955;41:849–3.

27. Burnet FM. The clonal selection theory of acquired immunity. London: Cambridge University Press; 1959.

28. Burnet FM. Autoimmune disease. BMJ. 1959; 2: 645–50 and 720–5.

29. Knight J, Laing P, Knight A, Adams DD. Ling N R. Thyroid-stimulating autoantibodies usually contain only λ light chains: evidence for the forbidden clone theory. J Clin Endocrinol Metab. 1986;62:342–7.

30. Pinchera A, Ingbar SH, McKenzie JM, Fenzi GF, editors. Thyroid autoimmunity. New York: Plenum Press; 1987.

31. Adams DD, Knight A, Knight JG, Laing P. Graves' disease; a paradigm for autoimmunity. In: Pinchera A, Ingbar SH, McKenzie JM, Fenzi GF, editors. Thyroid autoimmunity. New York: Plenum; 1987. p 1–10.

32. Smith GP. Filamentous fusion phage: novel expression vectors that display cloned antigens on the virion surface. Science. 1985;228:1315–7.

33. Scott JK, Smith GP. Searching for peptide ligands with an epitope library. Science. 1990;249:386–90.

34. Adams DD. Thyroid-stimulating autoantibodies. Vitam Horm. 1980;38:119–203.

35. Lindstrom J, Shelton D, Fujii Y. Myasthenia gravis. Adv Immunol. 1988;42:233–84.

36. Saus J, Wieslander CM, Langeveld JPM, Quinones S, Hudson BG. Identification of the Goodpasture antigen as the alpha 3 (IV) chain of collagen IV. J Biol Chem. 1988;263:13374–80.

37. Roitt IM, Doniach D, Shapland C. Autoimmune phenomena in relation to gastric mucosa in human disease. In: Grabar P, Miescher PA, editors Immunopathology. IVth International Symposium. Schwabe: Basel; 1965. P. 314–324.

38. Adams DD. Systemic lupus erythaematosus: a simple concept of the pathogenesis and its genetic basis. In: Dawkins RL, Christiansen FT, Zilko PJ, editors. Immunogenetics in rheumatology. Amsterdam: Excerpta Medica; 1982. p. 242–3.

39. Boey ML, Colaco CB, Gharadi AE, Elkon KB, Loizou S, Hughes GRV. Thrombosus in systemic lupus erythaematosus: striking association with the presence of circulating lupus anticoagulant. BMJ. 1983;287:1021–3.

40. Exner T. Lupus anticoagulant. Today's. Life Sci. 1989;1:40–6.

41. Davis AE, Ziegler JB, Gelfand EW, Rosen FS, Alpers CA. Heteeogeneity of nephritic factor and its identification as an immunoglobulin. Proc Natl Acad Sci USA. 1977;74:3980–3.

42. Kaplan ME. Autoimmune haemolytic disease due to warm-reacting antibodies. In: Wyngaarden JB, Smith LM, editors. Textbook of Medicine. 17th ed. Saunders: Philadelphia; 1985. p. 908–10.

43. Marcus AJ. Idiopathic thrombocytopenic purpura. In: Wyngaarden JB, Smith LM, editors. Textbook of medicine. 17th ed. Saunders: Philadelphia; 1985. p. 1033–4.

44. Wilson C, Ebringer A, Ahmadi K, Wrigglesworth J, Tiwana H, Fielder M, Binder A, Ettelaie C, Cunningham P, Joannou C, Bansal S. Shared amino acid sequences between major histocompatibility complex class II glycoproteins, type XI collagen and proteus mirabilis in rheumatoid arthritis. Ann Rheum Dis. 1995;54:216–20.

45. Menard HA, El-Amine M. The calpain-calpastatin system in rheumatoid arthritis. Immunol Today. 1996;17:545–7.

46. Knight JG. Dopamine receptor-stimulating autoantibodies: a possible cause of schizophrenia. Lancet 1982;ii:1073–6.

47. Knight JG, Knight A, Pert CB. Is schizophrenia a virally-triggered anti-receptor autoimmune disease? In: Helmchen H, Henn FA, ediors. Biological Perspectives of Schizophrenia. New York: Wiley; 1987. p.107–27.

48. Potter SR, Bienenstock J, Goldstein S, Buchanan WW. Fibroblast growth factors in scleroderma. J Rheumatol. 1985;12:1129–35.

49. Xu W, Leroy EC, Smith EA. Fibronectin release by systemic sclerosis and normal dermal fibroblasts in response to TGF-β. J Rheumatol. 1991;18:241-246.

50. Gilliland BC. Systemic sclerosis. In: Braunwald E, Fauci AS, Kasper DL, Hauser S, Longo Di, Jameson JL. (eds.) Harrison's Principles of Internal Medicine. 15th ed. New York: McGraw-Hill; 2001;1937–1946.

51. Fallon MD, Schwamm HA. Paget's disease of bone. Pathology Annual 1989;24:Part 1:115–159

52. Williams DG, Peters DK. Glomerulonephritis and renal manifestations of systemic disease. In: Weatheral DJ, Ledingham JGG, Warrell DA, editors. Oxford textbook of medicine. 2nd ed. University Press: Oxford; 1987. p. 36–55.

53. Bisno AL. Rheumatic fever. In: Wyngaarden JB, Smith LM, editors. Textbook of Medicine. 17th ed. Saunders: Philadelphia; 1985. p. 1527–33.

54. Tagg JR, McGiven AR, Guthrie DA. Heart-reactive antibodies in rheumatic fever. Med J Australia. 1972;1:621–624.

55. Dienstag JL, Isselbacher KJ. Autoimmune hepatitis. In: Braunwald E, Fauci AS, Kasper DL, Hauser SL, Longo DL, Jameson JL, editors. Harrison's principles of internal medicine. 15th ed. McGraw-Hill: New York; 2001. p. 1750–2.

56. Williams GH, Dluhy RG. Disorders of the adrenal cortex. In: Braunwald E, Fauci AS, Kasper DL, Hauser SL, Longo DL, Jameson JL, editors. Harrison's principles of internal medicine. 15th ed. McGraw-Hill: New York; 2001. p. 2084–105.

57. Rubin E, Faber J. Primary biliary cirrhosis. In: Rubin E, Farber JL, editors. Pathology. 2nd ed. Lippincott: Philadelphia; 1994. p. 740–743.

58. Hauser SL, Goodkin GE. Multiple sclerosis and other demyelinating diseases. In: Braunwald E, Fauci AS, Kasper DL, Hauser SL, Longo DL, Jameson JL, editors. Harrison's principles of internal medicine. 15th ed. McGraw-Hill: New York; 2001. p. 2452–2461.

59. Banker BQ, Engel AG. The polymyosytis and dermatomyositis syndromes. In: Engel AC, Banker BQ, editors. Myology: basic and clinical. McCraw Hill: New York; 1986. p. 1385–1422.

Chapter 3
Genetics

The Familial Aggregation

Studies of families, including twins, show that autoimmune diseases are weakly inherited, with disease specificity, the Mendelian pattern being that of causation by multiple, co-dominant (expressed in the heterozygous state) genes with incomplete penetrance [1]. What genes are these? Before discussing this we need to describe the histocompatibility system.

Discovery of the Histocompatibility System

This started in cancer research. By the beginning of the 1900s, cancer researchers, trying to prevent and cure cancer in people, realized that it would be helpful to their studies to be able to keep tumours going beyond the death of the laboratory animal in which it arose. However, they found that transferred tumours often died. An exception occurred when Japanese waltzing mice were used [2]. These animals, which had been bred by fanciers for generations in the Far East, were popular because people were amused by their antics, whirling and head-tossing. This is now known to be due to an inner ear (vestibular apparatus) defect, caused by a gene that is recessive, leading the fanciers to produce an inbred strain of mice with the defect always present. It was found that a carcinoma from one of these mice grew in all the waltzing mice to which it was transplanted, but not in any other mice. With discovery of the immunity system, making antibodies to attack invading germs, people suspected that it was the immunity system that caused the transplanted tumours to die, by attacking antigens on the tumour. However, Haldane [3] correctly postulated that the immune attack was directed at allo-antigens, not tumour antigens. He predicted that antigenic differences, similar to blood group differences, exist in tissues other than blood, and that a tumour arising in a given tissue preserves the alloantigenic characteristics of its host. He further correctly speculated that the allo-antigens induce an immune response in a new host lacking them.

D. D. Adams and C. D. Adams, *Autoimmune Disease*, 33
SpringerBriefs in Public Health, DOI: 10.1007/978-94-007-6937-3_3,
© The Author(s) 2013

This was the first recognition of the histocompatibility system, which is essential for defence against virus infection, prevents allo-transplantation and influences risk of autoimmune disease, as described below.

The Major Histocompatibility Complex

Unlike the blood group antigens, A, B, O, on red blood cells, important for blood transfusions, the histocompatibility antigens are on the surface of **all** nucleated cells, including the white cells, the leukocytes, where they were discovered and named by Dausset and Svejgard the human leucocyte antigens (HLA) [4]. The genes for the HLA antigens are in the **major histocompatibility complex (MHC)**, situated on the short arm of chromosome 6 in man and on chromosome 17 in the mouse [5].

Involvement of the MHC in Autoimmune Disease

After Vladutiu and Rose [6] had discovered that the MHC influences the occurrence of autoimmune disease in mice, world-wide studies found weak 2–5 fold associations between various autoimmune diseases and specific HLA antigens, but in 1973 Schlosstein and Terasaki [7] found a 69-fold association between ankylosing spondylitis and the HLA antigen B27. This galvanised the medical world, setting up numerous research studies, well summarized by Tiwari and Terasaki in their comprehensive 1985 review of HLA and disease associations [8].

Functions of the Major Histocompatibility Complex

First function. Defence against virus disease.

One of the classical experiments of recent times is that of Zinkernagel and Doherty [9], who found that virus-infected cells extrude peptides from the virus into the Bjorkman groove of their major histocompatibility antigens, this combined viral-histocompatibility antigen on the cell surface being the target for attack by the defensive cytotoxic T cells. Adams [10] realised that the explosive speed of viral replication [11] necessitates this histocompatibility antigen involvement, which directs the cytotoxic T cell attack on to the surface of the infected cell, destroying the virus factory, rather than ineffectively being muffled by the myriad numbers of free virions, as shown in Table 3.1. This explains the Simonsen phenomenon [12], our having huge clones of cytotoxic T cells reactive with allo-histocompatibility antigens, which our immune system mistakes for viral peptides on host histocompatibility antigens.

Table 3.1 The Histocompatibility system exists for defence against virus infection [10]

1. The race between virus and cytotoxic T cell		
The contestants	Replication time	Progeny
Influenza virus	10 h [11]	1,000 virions
Cytotoxic T cell	18 h	2 T cells

The race	Virions	T cells	Virion/T cell ratio
Day 1	1	10^6	$1/10^6$
Day 2	$1 \times 1{,}000^{2.4}$	$10^6 \times 2^{1.3}$	$6/1$
Day 3	2.5×10^{14}	6.3×10^6	$10^7/1$
Day 4	4×10^{21}	1.6×10^7	$10^{14}/1$

The result: the virus wins, the patient dies

2. Consequences of the explosive speed of viral replication

Hence, cytotoxic T cell clones need to be

1. Large, preformed [12] (no time for expansion)
2. Specific for conjoint virus-MHC antigenic target, so as not to be muffled by the myriad numbers of free virions
3. This explains
1. Why allografts are rejected
2. The strength of allograft rejection, Simonsen phenomenon [12].
3. The need for the MHC restriction phenomenon, discovered by Zinkernagel and Doherty [9], the presentation of viral antigens to cytotoxic T cells on host histocompatibility antigens, so that the anti-viral immune attack is directed at the virus-infected cells, the virus factories.

Second function. Imposition of polymorphism on the immune repertoire.

We all differ in our immune response repertoires in negative image of our very polymorphic histocompatibility antigens. This diversity usually enables some members of a population to survive an epidemic infection, preventing whole populations from being wiped out.

Third function. Defence against autoimmune disease.

This defence is imperfect, HLA-B27, with 69-fold increased risk of ankylosing spondylitis being one of the worst instances and HLA-DR2 one of the most successful with 7.7-fold decreased risk of Type 1 Diabetes.

Ebringer, determining the amino acid sequences of bacterial surface antigens has explained how the histocompatibility antigens influence the risk of development of pathogenic forbidden clones, as described later.

We have reached the stage of seeing how Darwinian natural selection of reproductive advantage governs the specificity of MHC genes for maximum protection against prevailing pathogenic microbes associated with a minimum of autoimmune disease.

Fourth function. Provision of a gene haven for MHC Class III gene products.

For the innate immune system, which developed before the adaptive antigen-specific system, certain molecules including tumour necrosis factor, the complement components C2, C4 and B, and adrenocortical steroids, are vitally important and need protection from immune attack. This is provided by siting their genes in

Table 3.2 Immune response genes. The germline H and V genes provide the germline predispositions to the autoimmune diseases and the random element of the somatic mutations in the lymphocyte V genes causes incomplete penetrance.

	Chain	Chromosome
A. Providing the repertoire, the germline V genes		
Genes for B cell antigen receptors	Heavy (V,D,J)	14q32.3
	κ light (V,J)	2p12
	λ light (V,J)	22q11
Genes for T cell antigen receptors	α (V,J)	14q11-12
	β (V,D,J)	7q32-33
	γ (V,J)	7p15
	δ (V,D,J)	14q11-12
B. Adding new clones to the repertoire, somatic mutations in the V genes of multiplying lymphocytes		
C. Subtracting from the repertoire, the H (histocompatibility antigen) genes which delete nascent complementary clones		
Major	α (very polymorphic)	6p
Class I (A, B, C)	β-2 microglobulin	15
Class II (DP, DQ, DR)	β (very polymorphic)	6p
	α (less polymorphic)	6p
Erythrocyte alloantigens	A, B, O	9
	others	various
The H-Y antigen, expressed in Bjorkman grooves	Y	
Other minor H antigens expessed in Bjorkman grooves	various	

the centre of the MHC gene complex, so that they can constantly be associated with protective Class I and II alleles [1].

Benacerraf and McDevitt's Mistake

Benacerraf and McDevitt [13] thought that the histocompatibility antigen genes influence risk of autoimmune disease by being linked to a special set of immune response genes, but these genes have never been demonstrated and it is now clear that it is the histocompatibility antigen genes themselves that are the immune response genes (Table 3.2) [1].

Solution of the Genetics of Autoimmune Disease; The H Gene Theory

The Bielschowskys' discovery of autoimmune haemolytic anaemia in their New Zealand Black inbred strain of mice [14] led to the further discovery by Howie and Helyer [15] of lupus nephritis in (NZB x NZW) F1 hybrid mice. Realising that this autoimmune kidney disease, not present in either parent, must be caused by at least one gene from each of the parental strains, Knight and Adams made backcross and linkage studies, finding three genes for lupus nephritis [16], one from the NZB mice and two from the NZW mice. This has been confirmed, corrected and extended by Drake et al. [17] and Kono et al. [18], using the wonderfully detailed microsatellite gene markers. In a similar study of the autoimmune anaemia of the NZB mice, using crosses with the NZC strain, a gene necessary for production of the anti-erythrocyte autoantibodies was found to be distantly linked to the black-brown coat colour gene on chromosome 4. In all, Knight and Adams found four genes, with linkage information coding for autoimmune disease in mice [19]. None were the expected V genes, one was in the MHC and two appeared to be in the neighbourhood of the minor histocompatibility antigens, *Hh* and *H-18*.

This was an example of the Einstein-cited [20] "stumble right up against the thing" that enabled Adams and Knight to link the fields of transplantation genetics [21], immunology, and autoimmunity to arrive at the H gene theory.

The H Gene Theory of Inheritance of Autoimmune Disease

This states that histocompatibility antigen genes, major, minor and HY (the male sex antigen), together with the V (variable region) genes coding for antigen receptors on B and T lymphocytes, are the germ-line immune response genes, the genes that influence the risk of autoimmune disease [22].

The Alternative Clonal Development Concept

The H gene theory received general acceptance and wide admiration when delivered by John Knight to a distinguished audience at a Ciba Foundation Symposium in London in 1982 [23]. Microbes bear multiple antigens and different lymphocyte clones compete with each other for reactivity with them. If a high affinity clone for a microbial antigen is missing, a lower affinity one for another antigen on the microbe will be stimulated. In this way, new clones can be **added** to the immune repertoire by deletion of their higher-affinity competitors [1, 10]. Without this understanding of how clonal deletions can add new clones to the repertoire, the great histocompatibility researcher, GD Snell, reluctantly withheld the H gene theory in 1968 [24].

Confirmation at the Molecular Level

As described later, Ebringer has confirmed the H gene theory and alternative clonal development concept at the molecular level, with measurements of the amino acid sequences of antigens on bacteria that trigger autoimmune diseases.

Immune Response Genes

Table 3.2 lists the genes that govern the specificity of immune responses, indicating how they work.

A Fourth Gene Category for McKusick's Catalogue

In the light of the Forbidden Clone and H Gene theories, the genetics of autoimmune disease changes from mystery, to elegant simplicity [23]. The key is the random element imposed on the genesis of an autoimmune disease by the need for unlucky somatic mutations in lymphocyte V genes. This explains the 50 % discordance of monozygous twins, despite their identical germ-line genes. Table 3.3 shows that Autoimmune provides a Fourth Category of gene to go with Dominant, Recessive and Sex-linked in McKusick's Catalogue of Mendelian Inheritance in Man [5].

Schizophrenia

As a medical student, in the 1940s, Adams was excited to be going into a mental hospital to learn about what he expected to be the myriad ways in which our complex brains could malfunction. However, to his surprise, the great majority of the patients were extraordinarily similar. Labelled "schizophrenics," they were preoccupied, often heard voices, like the French heroine Joan of Arc, often complained that a force was acting on them. In some patients the force was the Devil, in others, "wireless waves," in the early days of radio, then "atomic radiation," after advent of the atomic bomb. It was apparent to Adams that this meant that schizophrenia is not caused by any emotional upset, but is due to an acquired defect of biochemical activity in some part of the brain. The extremely limited and consistent nature of the abnormality was most encouraging, indicating causation by an acquired, precise defect of function and so giving great hope for the possibility of developing cure or prevention.

Table 3.3 A 4th Gene Category for McKusick's catalogue of Mendelian Inheritance

1. Dominant. Presence of the gene causes disease
2. Recessive. Absence of the gene causes disease
3. X-linked. Sex-linked. Gene on X chromosome
4. Autoimmune. Multiple co-dominant genes (V genes and H genes) with incomplete penetrance (due to need for antigenic triggers and somatic gene mutations in lymphocytes.) [22, 24]

The Knight Model of Schizophrenia

Working on Graves' disease, John Knight (Fig. 3.1) realized that schizophrenia has many similar aetiological features [25, 26]. Accordingly, he postulated that forbidden clones of B lymphocytes develop by somatic mutation, and make autoantibodies that act on neuronal cell receptors to affect the function of the brain's limbic system. Knight proposed that:

The familial aggregation is due to H genes and V genes.

The wait for V gene mutation explains the 50 % discordance of monozygous twins and the juvenile grace gap (relative absence in children).

Also explained are:

1. Seymore Kety' s adoptive studies showing a genetic basis for schizophrenia [27].
2. Remission and relapse.
3. The rheumatoid arthritis/schizophrenia discordance [28].

Furthermore, Harrison and Owen [29], reviewing genes predisposing to schizophrenia, in ignorance of the autoimmune model, found that there is evidence for involvement of chromosomal loci at three **immune response gene regions** (Table 3.2), namely 6p for the MHC, 22q11, spot on for λ immunoglobulin light chains, and chromosome 2, the site of κ light chains. This is powerful genetic evidence for the autoimmune model of schizophrenia.

The Knight model has no peer as an explanation of the pathogenesis and genetics of schizophrenia [30]. Discovery of its microbial trigger would enable prophylaxis of schizophrenia by vaccination against the microbe.

The recent demonstration that prednisone therapy lowers thyroid-stimulating autoantibody levels in Graves disease [31], suggests that its careful use [32] could be helpful in the therapy of schizophrenia, as it is in so many other autoimmune

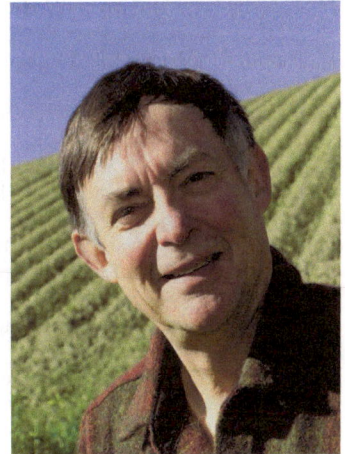

Fig. 3.1 Dr John G Knight, BSc (Hons) PhD. Disproved loss of suppressor T cells as the cause of autoimmunity in NZB mice. Proved forbidden clone theory for Grave's disease with measurement of κ and λ light chains. With DDA solved inheritance of autoimmune disease with H Gene theory. Author of the Knight model (autoimmune) of schizophrenia

diseases [33]. Immune ablation with stem cell rescue, as described below, with fortuitous timing, could prevent psychiatric disasters such as those at Port Arthur in Tasmania, Aramoana in New Zealand and Oslo in Norway.

Alan Ebringer's discovery of microbial triggers for rheumatoid arthritis and ankylosing spondylitis, described below, shows the urgent need for discovery of a microbial trigger for schizophrenia, which would enable **prophylaxis** of the disease by vaccination against its triggering microbe.

References

1. Adams DD, Knight JG. Principles of autoimmune disease: pathogenesis, genetics and specific immunotherapy. J Clin Lab Immunol. 2003;52:1–22.
2. Klein J. Biology of the mouse histocompatibility-2 complex. Berlin: Springer; 1975.
3. Haldane JBS. The genetics of cancer. Nature. 1933;132:265–7.
4. Dausset J, Svejgaard A. HLA and disease. Copenhagen: Munksgaard; 1977.
5. McKusick VA. Mendelian inheritance in man. 5th ed. Baltimore: Johns Hopkins University Press; 1978.
6. Vladutiu AO, Rose NR. Autoimmune mouse thyroiditis. Relation to histicompatibility type. Science. 1972;174:1137–8.
7. Schlosstein L, Terasaki PI, Bluestone R, Pearson GM. High association of an HL-A antigen, W27, with ankylosing spondylitis. N Engl J Med. 1973;288:704–6.
8. Tiwari JL, Terasaki PI. HLA and disease associations. New York: Springer; 1985.
9. Zinkernagel RM, Doherty PC. Restriction of in vitro T cell-mediated cytotoxicity in lymphocytic choriomeningitis within a syngeneic or semi-allogeneic system. Nature. 1974;248:701–2.
10. Adams DD. Protection from autoimmune disease as the third function of the major histocompatibility gene complex. Lancet. 1987; ii: 245–9.
11. Fenner F, White DO. Medical virology. London: Academic Press; 1975
12. Simonsen N. On the nature and measurement of antigenic strength. Transplant Rev. 1970;3:22–35.
13. Benacerraf B, McDevitt HO. The histocompatibility-linked immune response genes. Science. 1972;175:273–9.
14. Bielschowsky M, Helyer BJ, Howie JB. Spontaneous haemolytic anaemia in mice of the NZB/BL strain. Proc Univ Otago Med Sch. 1959;37:9–11.
15. Howie JB, Helyer BJ. The immunology and pathology of NZB mice. Adv Immunol. 1968;9:215–66.
16. Knight JG, Adams DD. Three genes for lupus nephritis in NZB × NZW mice. J Exp Med. 1978;147:1653–60.
17. Drake CG, Babcock SK, Palmer E, Kotzin EL. Genetic analysis of the NZB contribution to lupus-like autoimmune disease in (NZB × NZW) F1 mice. Proc Natl Acad Sci USA. 1994;91:4062–6.
18. Kono DH, Burlingame RW, Owen DG, Kuramochi A, Dalderas RS, Balomenos, D, Theofilopoulos, AN. Lupus susceptibility loci in New Zealand mice. Proc Natl Acad Sci USA 1994; 91:10168–72sss.
19. Knight JG, Adams DD. Genes determining autoimmune disease in New Zealand mice. J Clin Lab Immunol. 1981;5:165–70.
20. Einstein A. Essays in science. New York: Philosophical Library Inc; 1934. p. 92.
21. Auchincloss H, Sykes M, Sachs DH. Transplantation immunology. In: Paul WE, editor. Fundamental immunology. 4th ed. Philadelphia: Lippincott-Raven; 1999. p. 1175–235.

22. Adams DD, Knight JG. The H gene theory of inherited autoimmune disease. Lancet. 1980; i:396–8.
23. Knight JG, Adams DD. The genetic basis of autoimmune disease. Ciba Found Symp. 1982;90:35–56.
24. Snell GD. The H2 locus of the mouse: observations and speculations concerning its comparative genetics and its polymorphism. Folia Biol (Praha). 1968; 14:335–8.
25. Knight JG. Dopamine receptor-stimulating autoantibodies: a possible cause of schizophrenia. Lancet. 1982; ii:1073–6.
26. Knight JG, Knight A, Pert CB. Is schizophrenia a virally-triggered anti-receptor autoimmune disease? In: Helmchen H, Henn FA, editors. Biological perspectives of Schizophrenia. New York: Wiley; 1987. p. 107–27.
27. Kety SS. Mental illness in the biological and adoptive relatives of schizophrenic adoptees: findings relevant to genetic and environmental factors in etiology. Am J Psych. 1983;140:720–7.
28. Mellsop GW, Koadlow L, Syme J, Whittingham S. Absence of rheumatoid arthritis in schizophrenia. Aust N Z J Med. 1974;4:247–52.
29. Harrison PJ, Owen MJ. Genes for schizophrenia? Recent findings and their pathophysiological implications. Lancet 2003;361:417–9.
30. Gelder M, Gath D, Mayou R, Cowan P. Oxford Textbook of Psychiatry. 3rd ed. Oxford: Oxford University Press. 1998. p. 74–104.
31. Adams DD, Knight JG, Manning P, Smith G. An informative case of Graves' disease with implications for schizophrenia. J Clin Lab Immunol 2005;53:13–25.
32. Knight JG, Menkies DB, Highton J, Adams DD. Rationale for a trial of immunosuppressive therapy in acute schizophrenia. Molecular Psychiatry. 2007;12:421–31.
33. Kasper DL, Fauci AS, Longo DL, Braunwald E, Hauser SL, Jameson JL. (eds) Harrison's Principles of Internal Medicine 16th ed. New York: McGraw-Hill, 2005.

Chapter 4
Microbial Triggers

Rheumatic carditis and streptococci. Before the advent of penicillin, rheumatic fever with lesions of the heart and joints was a frequent autoimmune complication of infections by β-haemolytic streptococci of Lancefield Group A. This was because of an antigenic similarity between components of the streptococcus and heart tissue, found by Kaplan and Meyeserian [1]. Today, with such infections therapeutically aborted by penicillin, rheumatic heart disease, once common, has virtually disappeared in Western countries.

Glomerulonephritis and streptococci. Post-infective glomerulonephritis follows infection by Group A streptococci of multiple M types. This disease also is becoming less frequent due to use of antibiotics.

Reactive arthritis. This has been observed after enteric infection with *Shigella, Salmonella, Yersinia and Campylobacter* and genital infection with *Neisseria gonorrhea*.

Rheumatoid arthritis (RA) and *Proteus mirabilis* [2]. Multiple studies over three decades have found high titres of antibodies against this bacterium in a total of 1,375 RA patients, but not in other diseases or healthy controls, in studies by independent groups in 15 different countries. There was no such elevation in antibodies against 27 other microbial agents. There is evidence that the upper urinary tract is the main source of *Proteus* infection in RA (Fig. 4.1).

Ankylosing spondylitis (AS) and *Klebsiella* [3]. In world-wide studies involving 1330 AS patients and 1191 healthy controls, the AS patients showed significantly increased antibody titres to *Klebsiella*. There is evidence that the gut is the main site of *Klebsiella* infection in AS.

Schizophrenia and virus infection. Acute schizophrenia has been observed to follow upper respiratory tract virus infections and Knight has assembled much evidence indicating that schizophrenia is an autoimmune disease caused by autoantibodies that react with neuronal receptors influencing the limbic system [4, 5]. Seeking antigenic triggers and their corresponding autoantigen, with excellent technology at the NIH, Laing et al. immunized rabbits with neurotropic strains of influenza virus, inducing autoantibodies to a brain-specific 37-kDa

D. D. Adams and C. D. Adams, *Autoimmune Disease*,
SpringerBriefs in Public Health, DOI: 10.1007/978-94-007-6937-3_4,
© The Author(s) 2013

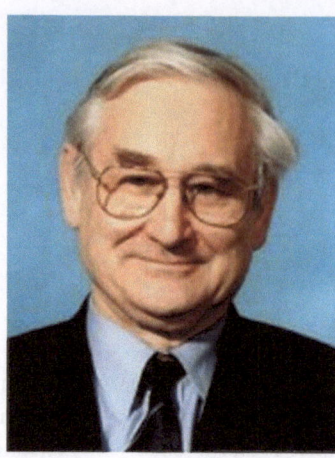

Fig. 4.1 Professor Alan Ebringer, BSc, MD, FRCP, FRACP. Discovered that *Proteus mirabilis* in the upper urinary tract triggers rheumatoid arthritis. Discovered that *Klebsiella pneumoniae* in the gut triggers ankylosing spondylitis. Confirmed the H gene theory by finding two antigens on *Proteus*, one resembling HLA-DR1/4 the predisposing HLA antigen, one resembling the autoantigen attacked. Showed how HLA-B27 predisposes, 69-fold, to ankylosing spondylitis

protein [6]. This needs further exploration, as does the whole field of psychotic aetiology, until the presumptive forbidden clones have been demonstrated with the clarity obtained for Graves' disease and myasthenia gravis.

Post-measles encephalomyelitis. This provided the first example of prophylaxis of an autoimmune disease by vaccination against its microbial trigger. Enders made a vaccine against measles, which rigorous studies by the National Communicable Disease Centre in Atlanta [7] showed gave 700-fold decreased risk of encephalomyelitis compared to the natural infection, as described below.

Information from Sequencing Antigens on Bacteria that Trigger Autoimmune Diseases

Details of the development of the methods used for successful determination of the amino acid sequences of antigens on the autoimmune disease-triggering bacteria, *Proteus mirabilis* and *Klebsiella pneumoniae,* are recorded in the book, "Rheumatoid arthritis and Proteus" by Alan Ebringer [8].

This research provides experimental confirmation, at the molecular level, of the H

Gene Theory of the inheritance of the autoimmune diseases, described above, by confirming the speculated presence of multiple antigens on triggering bacteria and alternative clonal development causing the autoimmune disease.

How Histocompatibility Antigens Predispose to Autoimmune Diseases

How HLA-DR1/4 predisposes to rheumatoid arthritis [3].

Figure 4.2 shows space-filling models of the amino acid sequences of the histocompatibility antigen, HLA-DR1/4 and the *Proteus mirabilis* haemolysin antigen. Close structural similarity is apparent. This means the immune tolerance imposed by the histocompatibility antigen will extend to this *Proteus* antigen, preventing immune reaction with it.

Figure 4.3 shows space-filling models of the amino acid sequences of the *Proteus mirabilis* urease antigen and Type 11 collagen, an autoantigen attacked in rheumatoid arthritis. The urease antigen is completely different from HLA-DR1/4, so will not be protected from immune reaction, being free to stimulate development of a forbidden clone reacting with the closely similar Type 11 collagen molecule, an autoantigen attacked in rheumatoid arthritis.

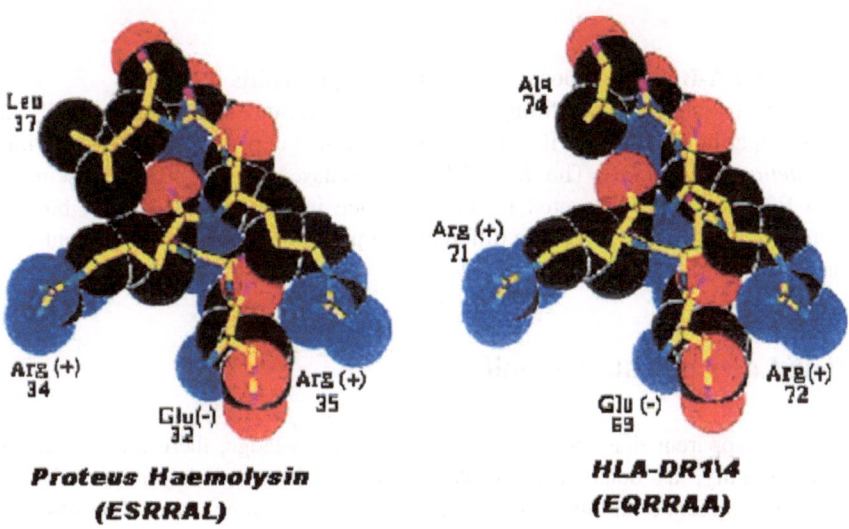

Fig. 4.2 Molecular similarity between histocompatibility antigen HLA-DR1/4 and *Proteus* haemolysin, preventing immune reaction against this bacterial antigen (Ebringer A. Rheumatoid Arthritis. Springer-Verlag, London. 2012)

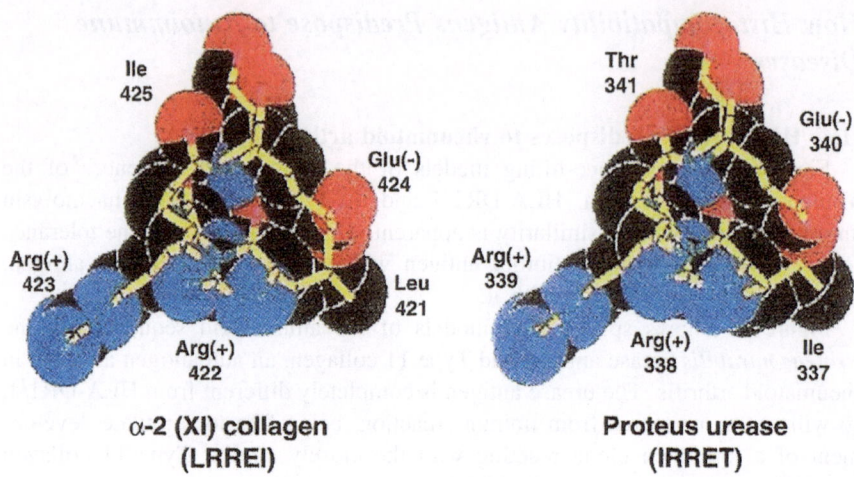

Fig. 4.3 Molecular similarity of *Proteus* urease and TypeXI collagen an autoantigen attacked in rheumatoid arthritis. This explains how infection with *Proteus mirabilis* causes rheumatoid arthritis (Ebringer A. Rheumatoid Arthritis. Springer-Verlag, London. 2012)

How HLA-B27 predisposes to ankylosing spondylitis [9].

Figure 4.4 shows space-filling models of the amino acid sequences of the histocompatibility antigen, HLA-B27 and two antigenic peptides on the bacterium *Klebsiella pneumoniae*. The *Klebsiella* nitrogenase antigen closely resembles HLA-B27, so will be covered by the tolerance induced by HLA-B27, but the bacterium's pullanase peptide is different and able to stimulate development of a forbidden clone, attacking the spine to cause causing ankylosing spondylitis.

Four Laws of Autoimmunity

It is now apparent that, in the present state of knowledge, there are 4 Laws of Autoimmunity, as detailed in Table 4.1. Recognition of the universality of microbial triggers of autoimmune diseases is a major advance, as it shows that all autoimmune diseases are potentially preventable by vaccinations against their microbial triggers, once these have been identified.

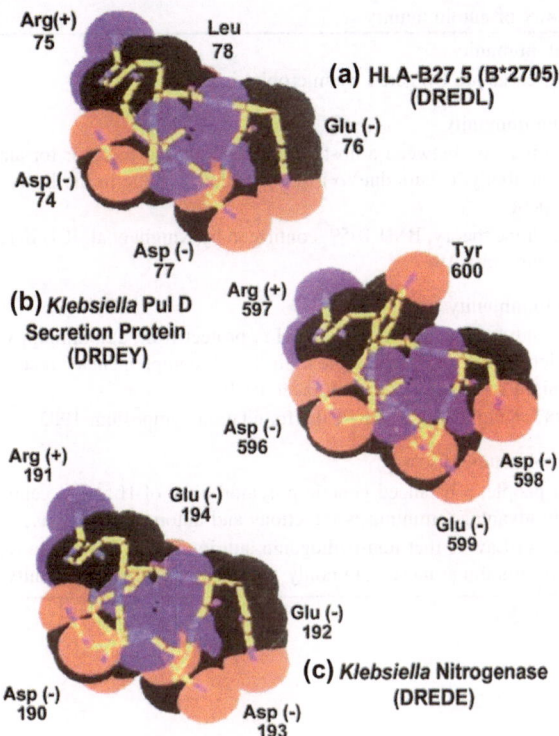

Fig. 4.4 Molecular similarity of HLA-B27 and the *Klebsiella nitrogenase* bacterial antigen, preventing immune reactivity, but dissimilarity with the *Klebsiella* pullonase bacterial antigen, allowing immune reactivity which can lead to development of the forbidden clones that cause ankylosing spondylitis, explaining the strong genetic predisposition (69-fold) by HLA-B27 discovered by Terasaki (Adams DD, Knight JG, Ebringer A. Autoimmune diseases. Autoimmunity Reviews 2010; 9: 525–530)

Table 4.1 Four laws of autoimmunity

The 1st law of autoimmunity
All autoimmune diseases are triggered by microbial infections
The 2nd law of autoimmunity
Autoimmunity, the reaction between a host component and the receptor for antigen on a lymphocyte or antibody, occurs due to a semi-random change in the DNA sequence of a lymphocyte V gene
Burnet's forbidden clone theory, BMJ 1959, confirmed by Knight et al. JCEM 1986, Adams et al. in thyroid autoimmunity 1987
The 3rd law of autoimmunity
Histocompatibility antigens, major, minor and HY, protect from autoimmunity with imperfect success, by deleting nascent lymphocyte clones with complementary receptors for antigen. Adams and Knight's H Gene Theory, Lancet 1980
Adams Lancet 1987, Knight and Adams Ciba foundation symposium 1982
The 4th law of autoimmune disease
In a population of people, a balanced genetic polymorphism of H and V genes, driven bt reproductive disadvantage, minimises infectious and autoimmune diseases
A corollary of the 4th Law is that non-pathogenic autoimmunity, having no reproductive disadvantage, occurs much more commonly than pathogenic autoimmunity

References

1. Kaplan MH, Meyeserian M. An immunological cross-reaction between group A streptococcal cells and human heart tissue. Lancet 1962;i:706–10.
2. Rashid T, Ebringer A. Rheumatoid arthritis is linked to Proteus—the evidence. Clin Rheumatol 2007;26:1036-43.
3. Wilson C, Ebringer A, Ahmadi K, Wrigglesworth J, Tiwana H, Fielder M, Binder A, Ettelaie C, Cunningham P, Joannou C, Bansal S. Shared amino acid sequences between major histocompatibility complex class II glycoproteins, type XI collagen and proteus mirabilis in rheumatoid arthritis. Ann Rheum Dis. 1995;54:216–20.
4. Knight JG. Dopamine receptor-stimulating autoantibodies: a possible cause of schizophrenia. Lancet 1982;ii:1073–6.
5. Knight JG, Knight A, Pert CB. Is schizophrenia a virally-triggered anti-receptor autoimmune disease? In: Helmchen H, Henn FA, ediors. Biological Perspectives of Schizophrenia. New York: Wiley; 1987. p.107–27.
6. Laing P, Knight JG, Hill JM, Harris JG, Webster RG et al. Influenza viruses induce autoantibodies to a brain-specific 37-kDa protein in rabbit. Proc Natl Acad Sci USA 1989;86:1998–2002.
7. National Communicable Disease Centre, Measles Surveillance. Report No. 7. Public Health Service, Atlanta.
8. Ebringer A. Rheumatoid arthritis and proteus. London: Springer; 2011.
9. Ebringer A, Rashid T, Wilson C, Ptaszynska T, Fielder M. Ankylosing spondylitis, HLA-B27, and Klebsiella pneumoniae—an overview proposed for early diagnosis and treatment. Curr Rheumatol Rev. 2006;2:55–68.

Chapter 5
Immunotherapy

Generalised Immune Suppression

Prednisone is judiciously used, short-term in high dosage and in low dosage for longer term, in the management of various autoimmune diseases [1], including the dangerous vasculitidies and sight-threatening exophthalmos.

Rituximab, is a monoclonal antibody preparation that binds to B cells and depletes them. For B cell-mediated autoimmune diseases, it might prove a useful alternative to prednisone and is in trial for systemic lupus erythematosus [2]. Some variants of rheumatoid arthritis might also be helped by rituximab, as Menard has found strong evidence that some cases are based on autoantibody destruction of calpastatin, which normally prevents intra-articular calpains from causing joint damage [3]. However, against the use of rituximab is the need for B cell activity for adequate immune defence against infection.

Immune Ablation and Autologous Bone Marrow Cell Restoration

Recently, Englert and her colleagues [4] saved the lives of three patients with systemic scleroderma of lethal severity. By destroying the patients' immune systems with immuno-suppressive chemotherapy, they got rid of their lethally-dangerous fibroblast-stimulating forbidden clones [5–7], then restored their immune systems with stem cells taken previously from each patient's own bone marrow. This autologous bone marrow grafting is necessary to prevent the patients from dying of microbial infections in the absence of their destroyed immunity systems [8]. Because forbidden clones of B or T lymphocyte cells arise by unlucky somatic mutations in their V genes, during the multiplication of lymphocytes in the periphery [9], they are very unlikely to reappear in the new, regenerated immune system. An alternative method for destroying the immune system would have been the use of total lymphoid irradiation [10]. This too would have destroyed the

D. D. Adams and C. D. Adams, *Autoimmune Disease*,
SpringerBriefs in Public Health, DOI: 10.1007/978-94-007-6937-3_5,
© The Author(s) 2013

forbidden clones of lymphocytes that were causing their patients' life-endangering systemic scleroderma.

As well as severe systemic scleroderma, other autoimmune diseases, in which immune system ablation followed by bone marrow rescue may be needed for severe cases, include rheumatoid arthritis, systemic lupus erythaematosis, myasthenia gravis, Goodpastures' syndrome and psychoses threatening suicide or murder.

Selective Destruction of Forbidden Clones

By far the best therapy for schizophrenia and other autoimmune diseases will be selective destruction of the pathogenic forbidden clones of lymphocytes, leaving the rest of the immune system intact. The research road towards this capability is now apparent [11]. It involves

1 *Finding the forbidden clones.* For seeking undiscovered ones, the receptor-ligand technology invented by GP Smith [12, 13] with patients' serum or cerebrospinal fluid screened on bacteriophage peptide display libraries, is a good way to seek pathogenic autoantibodies, and could be modified for seeking T cell forbidden clones, reactive with specific auto-antigens.
2 *Cloning the autoantigen.* After McLachlan and Rapoport [14] cloned thyroid peroxidase, the autoantigen for the thyroid microsomal autoantibodies, Vassart and Dumont et al. [15] cloned the TSH receptor, which is the autoantigen for Graves' disease. This has provided a autoantigenic molecule that is used for measuring the thyroid-stimulating autoantibodies [16].
3 *Attaching a cytotoxic moiety,* such as bungarotoxin or ^{131}iodine, emitting short-range beta particles, then administering the molecular complex intravenously to destroy the forbidden clones of plasma cells.

In Graves'disease itself, existing antithyroid therapy is good enough to make this new treatment unnecessary. However, for many other autoimmune diseases, especially schizophrenia, existing therapy is grossly unsatisfactory. It follows that there is an urgent research requirement for the development of technology that will enable the discovery of and specific destruction of the pathogenic forbidden clones.

Some lethal mysterious diseases, such as **multiple system atrophy** [17] may have an autoimmune basis, so their treatment by immune ablation and autologous bone marrow cell reconstitution, which is safe [10], should be explored.

References

1. Kasper DL, Fauci AS, Longo DL, Braunwald E, Hauser SL, Jameson JL. (eds) Harrison's Principles of Internal Medicine 16th ed. New York: McGraw-Hill, 2005.
2. Eisenberg R. Targeting B cells. In SLE; the experience with Rituximab treatment (anti-CD20). Endocrine, Metabolic and Immune Disorders Drug Targets. 2006;6:345–350.
3. Menard HA, El-Amine M. The calpain-calpastatin system in rheumatoid arthritis. Immunol Today. 1996;17:545–7.
4. Englert H, Katelaris C, McGill N, Schrieber L, Moore J. "Grape-sultana" sign represents a favourable response to aggressive treatment of early diffuse systemic scleroderma. Intern Med J. 2005;35:436–7.
5. Potter SR, Bienenstock J, Goldstein S, Buchanan WW. Fibroblast growth factors in scleroderma. J Rheumatol. 1985;12:1129–35.
6. Xu W, Leroy EC, Smith EA. Fibronectin released by systemic sclerosis and normal dermal fibroblasts in response to TGF-β. J Rheumatol 1991;18:241–246.
7. Gilliland BC. Systemic sclerosis. In: Braunwald E, Fauci AS, Kasper DL, Hauser S, Longo Di, Jameson JL. (eds.) Harrison's Principles of Internal Medicine. 15th ed. New York: McGraw-Hill; 2001;1937–1947.
8. Applebaum FR. Hematopoietic cell transplantation. In: Kasper DL, Fauci AS, Longo DL, Braunwald E, Hauser SL, Jamison JL. (eds.) Harrison's Principles of Internal Medicine. 16th ed. New York: McGraw-Hill; 2005;668-673.
9. Adams DD, Knight JG. Principles of autoimmune disease: pathogenesis, genetics and specific immunotherapy. J Clin Lab Immunol. 2003;52:1–22.
10. Fisher AJ, Rutherford RM, Bossino J, Parry G, Dark JH, Corris PA. The safety and efficacy of total lymphoid irradiation in progressive bronchiolitis obliterans syndrome after lung transplantation. American J Transplant 2005;5:537–534.
11. Adams DD. Seven deficiencies in Harrison's 16th edition 2005. J Clin Lab Immunol. 2006;54:1–13.
12. Smith GP. Filamentous fusion phage: novel expression vectors that display cloned antigens on the virion surface. Science. 1985;228:1315–7.
13. Scott JK, Smith GP. Searching for peptide ligands with an epitope library. Science 1990;249:386–390.
14. McLachlan SM, Rapoport B. The molecular biology of thyroid peroxidase: cloning, expression and role as an autoantigen in autoimmune thyroid disease. Endocrine Reviews 1992;13:192–206.
15. Perret J, Ludgate M, Libert F, Vassart G, Dumont J, Parmentier M. Stable expression of the human TSH receptor in CHO cells and characterisation of differentially expressing clones. Biochem Biophys Res Com. 1990;171:1044–50.
16. Costagliola S, Morgenthaler N, Hoemann K, Badenhoop K, Dumont J, Vassart G, et al. Second generation assay for TSH receptor antibodies has superior diagnostic sensitivity for Graves; disease. J Clin Endocrinol Metab. 1999;84:90–7.
17. Wenning GK, Stephania N. Recent developments in multiple system atrophy. J Neurol. 2009;. doi:10.1007/s00415-5173-8.

Chapter 6
Prophylaxis

Post-Measles Encephalomyelitis and Ender's Measles Vaccine

Following measles infection, encephalomyelitis occurs with a frequency of 1 in 1,000 cases [1]. After JF Enders produced a vaccine against measles, the National Communicable Disease Centre made rigorous study of the frequency of encephalomyelitis, following the natural infection and following vaccination with Ender's vaccine. They found that encephalomyelitis was 700 times more frequent after the natural infection than after the vaccine [2]. The vaccine must lack an antigen present on the measles virus, that triggers post-measles encephalomyelitis.

This was the first clear example of how vaccination against a microbial infection can prevent the autoimmune disease it triggers.

The Poliomyelitis Epidemics

A New Zealand example occurred in 1938, reported in the press and observed by Adams, trapped in a boarding school at the town of Masterton. An epidemic of leg paralyses occurred in Christchurch and spread progressively north, from town to town, to Picton, Wellington, Featherstone, then Carterton, the town next to Masterton, engendering great fear. Then, the boy in the bed next to Adams, complained of a stiff neck, was taken away, and reported to have polio. Six months later he returned with a paralysed leg. Adams and his other 30 school-mates were all unaffected.

D. D. Adams and C. D. Adams, *Autoimmune Disease*,
SpringerBriefs in Public Health, DOI: 10.1007/978-94-007-6937-3_6,
© The Author(s) 2013

Was the Paralysis a Rare Autoimmune Complication of Universal Virus Infection?

These events make it probable that the leg paralyses of poliomyelitis were a rare autoimmune complication of virtually universal virus infection, the paralyses probably caused by forbidden clones of cytotoxic T cells which attacked anterior horn neurons, hence the pathologists' name, "acute anterior poliomyelitis".

The Lead in Prophylaxis Given by the Polio Vaccines

The Salk (killed) and Sabin (attenuated) polio vaccines have both been brilliantly successful in preventing the polio leg paralyses. This exemplifies how autoimmune diseases in general, can be prevented by finding and vaccinating against their microbial triggers.

Finding Microbial Triggers

Ebringer has succeeded in this with rheumatoid arthritis [3] and ankylosing spondylitis [4], He has pioneered this new field of medical research, developing a whole new technology which needs to be copied in other diseases, especially schizophrenia. Systematic studies of other autoimmune diseases, with collaboration between clinicians and microbiologists are needed. The American Academy of Microbiology would be an ideal organizations for providing this urgently-needed knowledge.

Possible Therapy by Vaccination against Microbial Triggers

If vaccination against its microbial trigger has therapeutic effect on an autoimmune disease, it will be a major contribution to therapeutics. With present knowledge from Ebringer, this could be tested by vaccination against *Proteus mirabilis* for rheumatoid arthritis and vaccination against *Klebsiella pneumoniae* for ankylosing spondylitis.

A great objective will be to find the microbial trigger (probably viral) of schizophrenia, which currently lacks effective therapy.

The whole population cannot be vaccinated against every autoimmune disease, but with a 70-fold increased risk, males with HLA B27 are obvious candidates for vaccination against *Klebsiella pneumoniae*, to prevent their ankylosing spondylitis and to set the ball rolling.

References

1. Hauser SL, Goodkin GE. Multiple sclerosis and other demyelinating diseases. In: Braunwald E, Fauci AS, Kasper DL, Hauser SL, Longo DL, Jameson JL, editors. Harrison's Principles of Internal Medicine. 15th ed. McGraw-Hill: New York; 2001. p. 2452–61.
2. National Communicable Disease Centre, Measles Surveillance. Report No.7. Public Health Service, Atlanta.
3. Ebringer A, Rashid T, Wilson T, Ptaszynska T, Fielder M. Ankylosing spondylitis, HLA-B27, and Klebsiella—an overview: proposal for early diagnosis and treatment. Curr Rheumatol Rev. 2006;2:55–68.
4. Wilson C, Ebringer A, Ahmadi K, Wrigglesworth J, Tiwana H, Fielder M, Binder A, Ettelaie C, Cunningham P, Joannou C, Bansal S. Shared amino acid sequences between major histocompatibility complex class II glycoproteins, type XI collagen and proteus mirabilis in rheumatoid arthritis. Ann Rheum Dis. 1995;54:216–20.

Chapter 7
Transplantation

The histocompatibility system is responsible for the rejection of allografts. The system exists to counter the explosive speed of viral replication (Table 3.1). It does this by directing the defensive immune attack by cytotoxic T cells on to histo-compatibility antigens that have been altered by extrusion of a viral peptide on the infected cell's surface [1]. This enables destruction of the virus factories that the infected cells become, before the cytotoxic T cells are swamped by the myriad numbers of new virions, a thousand coming from each infected cell every 10 h in influenza infection [2]. The immunity system mistakes alloantigens for virus-infected host cells that need swift destruction.

Henry Kaplan, who revolutionised the treatment of Hodgkin's disease [3], found that animals could be made chimeras, by destroying their T and B lymphocytes by total lymphoid irradiation, followed by inoculation with allogeneic bone marrow, after which they could accept allogeneic skin and organ grafts from the donor of the bone marrow [4].

Megan Sykes [5] has improved Kaplan's technique by adding recipient bone marrow cells to the donor ones injected for reconstitution of the recipient after immune ablation.

As Adams [6] emphasises, this protocol is in urgent need of application, as it would enable **xenografting from untreated pigs**, offering instant and unlimited supply of grafts for man, transforming the presently unsatisfactory field of transplant surgery.

Acknowledgments We are indebted to Pro-Vice-Chancellor, Peter Crampton for encouragement, information, advice and administrative support.

References

1. Zinkernagel RM, Doherty PC. Restriction of in vitro T cell-mediated cytotoxicity in lymphocytic choriomeningitis within a syngeneic or semi-allogenic system. Nature. 1974; 248: 701–702.
2. Fenner F, White DO. Medical virology. London: Academic Press; 1975.

3. Kaplan HS. Hodgkin's disease: unfolding concepts concerning its nature, management and prognosis. Cancer. 1980;45:2439–74.
4. Slavin S, Reitz B, Bieber C, Kaplan HS, Strober S. Transplantation tolerance in adult rats using total lymphoid irradiation; permanent survival of skin, heart and marrow allografts. J Exp Med. 1978;147:700–7.
5. Sykes M. Mixed chimerism and transplant tolerance. Immunity. 2001;14:417–24.
6. Adams DD. Why the histocompatibility system exists and how transplant surgeons can xenograft without rejection. Q J Med. 2011;104:767–9.